Applied Health Humanities for the Aging

This book provides a collection of interventions from researchers' and clinicians' health humanities experiences, and makes their methods available to home and institutional caregivers to aid interactions with the elderly, particularly persons diagnosed with dementia.

As a revolutionary perspective connecting medical training and treatment with lessons from the humanities, medical humanities emphasizes the treatment and care of disease, the "science of the human," and offers an integrated approach to health professional education that include lessons from comparative religion, history, literature, philosophy, the visual and performing arts.

Highlighting the needs of persons with dementia and their caregivers, this compilation shows how the arts can play a primary role in empowering families and communities to offer creative and meaningful care within their own homes and communities. Each chapter provides an overview of a specific creative application (reading and commonplacing; storytelling; intergenerational musical activities; Bingocize®; haiku making; and animatronic pet activities), the evidence-based support for its benefits, and clear and accessible instructions for the reader. These methods offer insightful approaches to care in which skills such as active listening can provide in-roads to patient experiences as well as an array of creative approaches to ameliorate the physical and mental consequences of isolation and loneliness that too often accompany aging and disease.

This text will be of interest to healthcare workers and allied health professionals, healthcare administrators and family members.

Trini Stickle, PhD, is an applied linguist at Western Kentucky University. She primarily focuses on factors that negatively affect persons' access to meaningful interaction, including individuals diagnosed with dementia or autism and English language learners. Her work identifies barriers unique to each group and the strategies needed to overcome these difficulties. Stickle is also investigating the aging experiences of immigrant and refugee populations living in southern regions of the US.

Lorna E. Segall, PhD, MT-BC, is associate professor and director of music therapy at the University of Louisville. Her research and project development explores intergenerational programming and music in prisons. Additionally, she engages her students in this work in an effort to promote understanding, compassion and humanizing with respect to often misunderstood and underserved populations.

Applied Health Humanities for the Aging

Activities for Home and Institutional Caregivers

Edited by Trini Stickle and
Lorna E. Segall

Routledge
Taylor & Francis Group

LONDON AND NEW YORK

Designed cover image: Getty image number 1353055997

First published 2025
by Routledge
4 Park Square, Milton Park, Abingdon, Oxon OX14 4RN

and by Routledge
605 Third Avenue, New York, NY 10158

Routledge is an imprint of the Taylor & Francis Group, an informa business

© 2025 selection and editorial matter, Trini Stickle and Lorna E. Segall; individual chapters, the contributors

The right of Trini Stickle and Lorna E. Segall to be identified as the authors of the editorial material, and of the authors for their individual chapters, has been asserted in accordance with sections 77 and 78 of the Copyright, Designs and Patents Act 1988.

British Library Cataloguing-in-Publication Data
A catalogue record for this book is available from the British Library

Library of Congress Cataloging-in-Publication Data
Names: Stickle, Trini, editor. | Segall, L. (Lorna), editor.
Title: Applied health humanities for the aging : activities for home and
   institutional caregivers / edited by Trini Stickle and Lorna E. Segall.
Description: Abingdon, Oxon ; New York, NY : Routledge, 2025. |
   Includes bibliographical references and index.
Identifiers: LCCN 2024032199 (print) | LCCN 2024032200 (ebook) |
   ISBN 9781032417288 (hardback) | ISBN 9781032417271 (paperback) |
   ISBN 9781003359463 (ebook)
Subjects: LCSH: Older people—Care. | Dementia—Patients—Care. |
   Medicine and the humanities.
Classification: LCC HV1451 .A695 2025 (print) | LCC HV1451 (ebook) |
   DDC 362.6—dc23/eng/20241118
LC record available at https://lccn.loc.gov/2024032199
LC ebook record available at https://lccn.loc.gov/2024032200

ISBN: 978-1-032-41728-8 (hbk)
ISBN: 978-1-032-41727-1 (pbk)
ISBN: 978-1-003-35946-3 (ebk)

DOI: 10.4324/9781003359463

Typeset in Sabon
by Apex CoVantage, LLC

We dedicate this book to the many individuals—old and young—who go through each day wishing they had someone with whom they might spend an hour to talk or walk, create a story or poem, sing or make music, share a memory, play a game—or, simply, be engaged.

Contents

Figures and Tables

Figures

Tables

Contributors

Charley Baker, PhD, School of Health Sciences, University of Nottingham, UK

Kaitlyn Beard, MM, MT-BC, CDP, NICU-MT, Big Bend Hospice, Tallahassee, Florida, US

Brian Brown, PhD, School of Applied Social Sciences, De Montfort University Leicester, UK

K. Jason Crandall, PhD, EP-C, School of Kinesiology, Recreation & Sport, Western Kentucky University, Bowling Green, Kentucky, US

Boyd H. Davis, PhD, applied linguistics, emerita, University of North Carolina–Charlotte, North Carolina, US

Jessica L. Folk, MFA, Potter College of Arts & Letters, Western Kentucky University, Bowling Green, Kentucky, US

Cameron Fontes, writer, Louisville, Kentucky, US

Gillian Knoll, PhD, Potter College of Arts & Letters, Western Kentucky University, Bowling Green, Kentucky, US

Dana Nguyen Le, neuroscience and psychology student, Vanderbilt University College of Arts and Sciences, Vanderbilt University, Nashville, Tennessee, US

Mackenzie Leighty, MT-BC, Music Speaks LLC, Madison, Wisconsin, US

Margaret Maclagan, PhD, School of Psychology, Speech and Hearing, retired, University of Canterbury, Canterbury, NZ

Harumi Maeda, Japanese linguistics doctoral candidate, Department of East Asian Languages and Cultures, Stanford University, California, US

Yoshiko Matsumoto, PhD, Department of East Asian Languages and Cultures, Stanford University, California, US

Caroline Mwende, MT-BC, music therapist, Cincinnati, Ohio, US

Debra Sheets, PhD, MSN, RN, FAAN, School of Nursing, Emerita & Institute on Aging and Lifelong Health, University of Victoria, British Columbia, CA

Victoria Tischler, PhD, School of Psychology, University of Surrey, Guildford, UK

Meredith Troutman-Jordan, PhD, PMHCNS-BC, School of Nursing, University of North Carolina–Charlotte, North Carolina, US

Emily Wan, doctoral candidate, Department of East Asian Languages and Civilizations, Harvard University, Boston, Massachusetts, US

Acknowledgements

We would like to express our appreciation to the following people.

Each contributor to this collection who has made this work a joy to watch come together. We have learned so much for each chapter, and we know others will greatly benefit as well.

We thank the many, generous participants of our collective research upon whose shoulders our work rests and from which the activities within the chapters were created.

We thank the Routledge team—Claire Jarvis, in particular—who were dedicated to seeing this work completed.

We thank our friends and colleagues who allowed us time and provided encouragement.

And, mostly, we thank our families who supported us by sacrificing their time with us, filling in the gaps when we needed time, and understanding how important this work is for us and for the many lonely people whose lives we hope are enriched and engaged through the activities described within these pages.

We also wish to celebrate the caregivers who give everything they have within their emotional and physical capacity to support the wellbeing of others without a word of praise or encouragement.

Abbreviations

ADLs	activities of daily living
AI	artificial intelligence
AIR	artist in residence
BIPOC	Black, indigenous, and other people of color
CDC	Center for Disease Control
CITI	Collaborative Institutional Training Initiative
CNA	certified nurse attendant
CORE	Companions of Respected Elders
COVID-19	coronavirus disease 2019
LGBTQIA+	people who identify as lesbian, gay, bisexual, transgender, queer (or questioning their gender), intersex, asexual and their allies.
MCI	mild cognitive impairment
MMSE	Mini Mental State Examination
NCCCH	National Commission on Correctional Health Care
NCOA	National Council on Aging
NIA	National Institutes on Aging
NIH	National Institutes of Health
PHSK	Presbyterian Homes and Services of Kentucky
PwD	persons with dementia or persons living with dementia
QoL	quality of life
ViM	Voices in Motion
WHO	World Health Organization

Part I

1 History and Applications of Health Humanities

Brian Brown, Charley Baker and Victoria Tischler

Introduction: The Histories and Potentials of Health Humanities

In this chapter, we outline the evolution of what was previously called the "medical humanities" into a broader focus on the "health humanities" and sketch out some of the implications and applications where older adults are concerned. The authors of this chapter have been involved closely in this shift in focus and have gained some insight over the years as to how this has come about and its current directions.

Medical Humanities

The story of the medical humanities and its role in medical education is well known. In addition to teaching the knowledge of and skills to treat disease and injury, medical education has drawn from the humanities by including courses on the ethics of patient care and treatment as well as on the history and philosophy of medicine. With a growing interest in patient experience and satisfaction, there came an expanded focus on the role of the arts and humanities in helping to create a more humane and empathetic mindset among physicians. Hence, efforts to include novels, plays, the cinema, music and the like into medical education began to proliferate. The notion was that through artifacts curated from the humanities, future clinicians would learn how better to treat *the person* rather than simply focusing on the disease or injury of *the patient*. The presence of medical humanities education expanded in many of the world's medical schools, initially in Europe and the United States. While the incorporation of medical humanities across medical schools did increase, many clinical and caregiver programs did not include these types of courses. Additionally, the full potential of the humanities as part of care and healing were not addressed within the "standard" medical humanities canon.

DOI: 10.4324/9781003359463-2

In one of our first publications, we attempted to remit the definition for this new field of medical humanities, going beyond the notion of simply educating clinicians through artifacts taken from the humanities and arguing for a "more inclusive, outward-facing and applied discipline, embracing interdisciplinarity and engaging with the contributions of those marginalized from the medical humanities" (Crawford et al., 2010, p. 4). Here, we sought to include perspectives from the wider public, as well as those groups variously called patients, clients, users, or others with "lived experience." Moreover, it was apparent to us that informal carers, allied health professionals such as nurses, occupational therapists and care assistants also had important perspectives to offer the humanities as did other members of the workforce in health, social and education settings. We also found that many of the diverse groups of caregivers were actually drawing upon their knowledge of the arts and humanities in their work, yet many were not, and still are not, being systematically taught using illustrations taken from the humanities in their coursework.

The value of arts and humanities activity for informal carers, for instance, were hardly mentioned in the literature. Seldom was attention given to the variety of paraprofessionals and support staff who contribute to the health care journey. For example, people who provide catering and cleaning services in hospitals may interact with patients and influence the emotional tone of the hospital stay. Yet, all this is virtually *terra incognita*, that is *unexplored territory,* as far as the research community is concerned. Likewise, despite their substantial contributions to health care delivery, paramedics, ambulance staff, physiotherapists, receptionists and members of charitable, or voluntary organizations are relatively unknown within the existing medical humanities literature, yet they are an integral part of many patient journeys. Importantly, then, was the turn to the humanities—its artifacts and practices—for the patient's, or more accurately, for the person's journey as part of the treatment and healing process.

Health Humanities

Expanding the use of artifacts and practices from medical education to a wide range of clinician and caregiver training and then to patient care led to the concept of health humanities. As Jones et al. (2017) state, adopting the term *health humanities* is not merely semantic or "splitting hairs." Given the range of subjects, health professions, stakeholders and practice environments involved, health humanities is a "more encompassing, contemporary, and accurate label" (Jones, 2014, p. 34).

This desire to incorporate more professions, perspectives and constituencies into the field has been a pervasive feature of our efforts to promote the idea of "health humanities" in the twenty-first century. As Crawford and Brown (2020) wrote more recently, the health humanities offer a "superordinate evolution" that advances innovation, mutuality and dialogue between congruent traditions. In this way, it seeks to inspire and facilitate rather than to govern innovation, education and care.

Among the possibilities of the heath humanities perspective, Charise states that "[o]ne of the innovations of health humanities is its radically interdisciplinary approach, which differs from conventional health education by foregrounding subjects that generally value aesthetics, social experiences, and interpretive methods over quantitative and/or biomedical modes of investigation" (2017, p. 433). She describes how health humanities can provide an open and diverse "undergraduate, pre- or non health-professional field of study," and more broadly, a "vibrant site of public learning and activism" (Charise, 2017, p. 444).

One of the features of our approach has been to initiate an epistemological shift. That is, it has been possible to mark out some changes concerning the nature and origins of knowledge. Previously, the arts were seen as additive; something that could be used to disseminate messages and conclusions from more conventionally conducted research, perhaps to enhance the public's "awareness" or "health literacy." In our approach, we have sought to bring to the forefront the possibilities of the arts and creative disciplines as methods of inquiry in their own right. This has been a feature of our work to take the health humanities into an international arena. For example, the work that we have done concerning mental health and resilience in India has used the medium of community theatre. For example, this has yielded unique insights concerning the nature of resilience among migrants in a low-income neighborhood (Raghavan et al., 2022a). The combination of theatre and music activities as well as arts and crafts provided a starting point for conversations that enriched the psychological concept of resilience by embedding it within social and familial contexts and showing how it was intertwined with memories of the past as well as the hopes of future generations.

In a further study concerned with mental health in Kerala (India), also using community theatre, we saw it was possible to reconceptualize ideas around mental health literacy. The construct is typically taken to denote the extent to which a person subscribes to the dominant medico-therapeutic ideas around mental health in the Global North. Yet, in our study, it became apparent that participants were literate in a variety of idioms of distress and healing, which encompassed social, familial and spiritual aspects of the problem. Rather than a single kind of thinking on the matter, there were multiple mental health literacies at work (Raghavan et al., 2022b). The integration of religious faith and spiritual awareness with notions of healing was profound. For some participants, it was the strength of their faith which was believed to make the "Western" treatments work at all (Raghavan et al., 2022c). Stigma in relation to mental health also was understood differently. Rather than being about individual prejudice, as it is often conceived in the Global North, in India it was apt to involve a variety of familial and community concerns, such as worries about the future marriageability and family life of the affected person (Raghavan et al., 2022d). Here, we see the healing power of the humanities can be directed toward the health of the greater society.

The point here is not to assert that our findings are veridical across all population groups—there may be important variations and local nuances as yet unexplored—but rather to underline the possibilities for interrogation and reconceptualization that arise if the arts-based methods are allowed stature as primary methods of inquiry. Instead of being tools to raise awareness of mental health or impose a particular medico-therapeutic view of the issue, the arts are fundamental to our opportunities for rethinking and re-evaluating some of the key concepts in health and wellbeing. Thus, a further concern and one germane to this volume is the use of the artifacts and practices of heath humanities as part of treatment: societal and individual.

Health Humanities and the Care of Older People

A similar argument can apply to the health humanities and the experiences of old age. For example, where music is concerned, Wood (2020) reminds us that in dementia care, music is recognised to have clinical and recreational value for its ability to help create meaning and facilitate relationships. However, it has yet "to be used as a core method of research for analyzing everyday speech or care interactions" (Wood, 2020, p. 76). Accordingly, in considering the interactions of carers and dementia patients as they go about everyday tasks like eating dinner, Wood elucidates the tone and rhythm of the interactions. Indeed, he talks about how musical categories of experience are co-created between people in dementia care settings. An approach which treats conversational interaction as if it were music enables us to see the interactional structures by which the people in the setting use to achieve a conversational to and fro, despite interruptions and simultaneous attempts to speak or long silences. This enables a richer understanding of the dance—if you will—of conversation, over and above what might be noticed simply by transcribing the words or checking their lexical meaning. Such an analysis, says Wood, enables us to capture the "characteristic phrasal patterns" (2020, p. 78) which might, in a mere transcript, look like it was disjointed or hard to understand. This might include unphrased speech, compact forms, broken or truncated phrases, monosyllabic utterances and repetition. These elements which become meaningful when considered part of the "music" of conversation persist and remain intelligible even where the speech involves non-standard grammar, or where words themselves are lost, compressed, or broken. Moreover, the patient's and carer's speech patterns, Wood describes, are imitative and convergent—people continue to engage in the "dance" of conversation even when one member's ability to produce words of the kind you find in a dictionary is impaired. In this example, adopting an arts and humanities-focused "frame" to understand the situation can yield fresh insights into how communication and social relationships can be sustained despite neurodegenerative problems making inroads into a person's capability.

These kinds of conceptual and philosophical considerations can have valuable implications for the care of people who may appear confused and disorientated. Williams and Zeilig (2023) consider the notion of agency—the feeling of ownership of one's actions and responsibility for them. This, they argue, can have multiple dimensions, involving embodiment, emotions, intentions and decision making. They provide an example of how an elderly woman with Alzheimer's disease was enabled to participate in a musical activity. While she did not initially respond when presented with a drum, after a short while she was tempted to tap out a rhythm while the music therapist held the drum for her. In the process of this, she was able to exchange smiles with other musicians in the session. What might initially seem to be a small change, this example shows how, even when in middle-to-late stage Alzheimer's disease, social relationships—and by implication the sense of self as a social being—can be enhanced. The creative disciplines offer opportunities for people nearing the end of life or who are experiencing neurodegenerative symptoms to be creative actors in their own right. A well-known case is that of the popular novelist Terry Pratchett (1948–2015). Pratchett lived with Alzheimer's disease for the last decade of his life, yet he continued writing until very shortly before his death, with his final writings being published posthumously. Less well-known is the case of Paul Watts who was living with dementia composed the inspiring piece of music *Four Notes* while "incapacitated" with the condition. As Oliver Sacks (2007) and many others have noted, the ability to appreciate and produce music can be remarkably robust in the face of challenges such as neurodegenerative conditions, head injuries and stroke.

A further challenge in delivering healthcare to older adults is the gulf that may exist between practitioners and those for whom they care. As students take courses to prepare them to be doctors, nurses, or other health care professionals, the people involved are likely to be young adults, barring the occasional mature student. Similarly, early in one's career, there is likely to be a good deal of patient-facing work. By contrast, patients nearing the end of their lives are likely to be elderly, with different histories, life experiences and priorities. Many of their significant life course waymarkers occurred before the health professionals treating them were born or, at least, cognizant of these important events. Bridging these experiential worlds may present a challenge. Here, too, arts- and humanities-based interventions may be used to address these experiential differences. For instance, McCaffrey et al. (2017) describe how his team attempted to deploy Joan Barfoot's novel *Exit Lines* in the education of nursing students working with older adults. The novel described patients in a similar facility to the one where the trainee nurses were working. McCaffrey et al. (2017) report how the novel enhanced the students' conceptual and interpretive flexibility in making sense of differing perspectives and ways of knowing when they interacted with older persons within their care. In this respect, the student clinicians appeared to become more self-aware and humane practitioners as clinicians.

Health Humanities and its Limitations

Despite many promising and exciting avenues for practice and research, there remain significant limitations to the health humanities. Despite our enthusiasm for welcoming the contributions of non-medical helping professionals and informal carers, these areas are still in need of development. A lingering hegemony, or, at a minimum, dominating thought, of medical categories exists, specifically for journal editors and reviewers who have a distinct preference for work focusing on people with a single diagnosable condition. They often criticize work that does not merely focus on a homogenous group who all have, say, depression or diabetes, which means that it is difficult to publish on the effects of these innovative approaches. Additionally, many studies using the health humanities within the field are still relatively small and exploratory. This gives us a great deal of reported "lived experience" information, yet there is still relatively little that demonstrates significant statistical advantages of arts and humanities focused work at large scale.

Health Humanities Potentials

These limitations aside, the health humanities have succeeded in creating a more inclusive, outward-facing, and applied field for the arts and humanities within patient care environments. Beyond simply medical education, health humanities contribute to the health and wellbeing of the public or social health, not least for those experiencing the isolating and debilitating effects of ageing. In the early days of our journey towards the health humanities, we were relatively few voices in comparison to the much better-established medical humanities. However, since we have been promoting the idea, it has become a much more widely used and, dare we say it, powerful phrase. It has found its way into the titles of courses, conferences, books, periodical literature and treatment methods. Perhaps the growing popularity of health humanities owes something to their egalitarian, co-productive and democratizing approach. In other words, they have become more powerful because there are so many more people who can contribute. Different professional groups, patients, service users, and those with lived experience, informal charitable and voluntary groups, and the interested general public can all contribute. Within the academic and professional sphere, it has enabled a critical meeting ground with related disciplines, traditions or missions, not least medical humanities, arts for health, arts therapies and the work of many different creative disciplines which have not hitherto been thought of in this way. Architecture, textiles and needlecraft, even horticulture are examples of this, where people are thinking more imaginatively and rigorously about the relation between places, spaces, craft activities and health, wellbeing and resilience. Some of these insights have a long pedigree, too. The nineteenth-century asylums in Britain were often designed to offer the latest in architecture, as well as activities such as gardening, farming, textile and needlecrafts. This is not to romanticize old-style custodial care or relentless toil in the asylum laundry, but rather to highlight the way that shared practical activity has long been believed to have benefits.

A creative life, even while living with dementia, is possible. This can be enhanced with the input of arts, health and social care professionals or family carers, yet it is even possible where formal professional input is absent. Persons living with dementia may already be utilizing cultural assets independently, advancing health and wellbeing for themselves or others through creative activities and performance despite illness or discomfort. The health humanities champion the agency of people who might otherwise be treated merely as patients or clients or are deemed mere recipients of professional healthcare interventions and values a more joyful and collaborative vision. Via the health humanities it is possible to challenge the framing of people living with dementia as merely having deficits, or being somehow lacking or incapable—that is, as resource depleted. The health humanities can bring a more mutual force into play, seeking new pathways to a less centralized "creative public health" (Crawford & Brown, 2020).

Conclusion

Ultimately, it may be possible to re-frame the contribution of the health humanities to health itself. Up to now, arts and humanities activities have often been used as if they were something that could be prescribed as a kind of therapeutic medicine, or something that could be used to disseminate or educate. Taken in their fullest sense, the health humanities can help us challenge these unidirectional approaches to the use of the arts and humanities, which see them as something that may be "injected" by experts into the frail and broken. It may be possible, via the arts and humanities, to achieve a genuine dialogue involving all parties. We expect the chapters that follow to help move this dialogue into its next, needed direction.

References

Charise, A. (2017). Site, sector, scope: Mapping the epistemological landscape of health humanities. *Journal of Medical Humanities*, *38*(4), 431–444.

Crawford, P., Brown, B., Tischler, V., & Baker, C. (2010). Health humanities: The future of medical humanities? *Mental Health Review Journal*, *15*(3), 4–10.

Crawford, P., & Brown, B. (2020). Health humanities: Democratising the arts and humanities applied to healthcare, health and wellbeing. In A. Bleakley (Ed.), *Handbook of medical humanities* (pp. 401–409). Routledge.

Jones, T. (2014). "Oh, the Humanit(ies)!" Dissent, democracy, and danger. In V. Bates, A. Bleakley, & S. Goodman (Eds.), *Medicine, health and the arts: Approaches to the medical humanities* (pp. 27–38). Routledge.

Jones, T., Blackie, M., Garden, R., & Wear, D. (2017). The almost right word: The move from medical to health humanities. *Academic Medicine*, *92*(7), 932–935.

McCaffrey, G., Venturato, L., Patterson, D., Langille, J., Jackson, R., & Rosenal, T. (2017). Bringing a novel to practice: An interpretive study of reading a novel in an undergraduate nursing practicum course. *Nurse Education in Practice*, *24*, 84–89, https://doi.org/10.1016/j.nepr.2017.04.001

Raghavan, R., Brown, B., Coope, J., Crossley, M., Sivakami, M., Gawde, N., Pendse, T., Jamwal, S., Barret, A., Dyalchand, A., Chaturvedi, S., Chowdary, A., & Heblikar, D. (2022a). Idioms of resilience: Mental health and migration in India. *International Journal of Social Psychiatry*, *68*(8), 1607–1613. https://doi.org/10.1177/00207640211042916.

Raghavan, R., Brown, B., Horne, F., Kamal, S. R., Parameswaran, U., Raghu, A., Wilson, A., Venkateswaran, C., Svirydzenka, N., Lakhanpaul, M., & Dasan, C. (2022b). Multiple mental health literacies in a traditional temple site in Kerala: The intersection between beliefs, spiritual and healing regimes. *Culture, Medicine and Psychiatry*, *47*(3), 743–765. https://doi.org/10.1007/s11013-022-09800-6

Raghavan, R., Brown, B., Hussain, S., Kumar, S., Wilson, A., Svirydzenka, N., Kumar, M., Ali, A., Chandrasekharan, A., Banu-Soletti, A., Lakhanpaul, M., Iyer, M., Venkateswaran, C., Dasan, C., Sivakami,

M., Manickam, S., Barrett, A., & Wilson, M. (2022c). How do Muslim service users, caregivers and community members in Malappuram, Kerala, use their faith to address the challenges associated with mental ill health? *Mental Health Religion and Culture, 25*(10), 1012–1025. https://doi.org/10.1080/13674676.2023.2169268.

Raghavan, R., Brown, B., Horne, F., Kumar, S., Parameswaram, U., Bin Ali, A., Raghu, A., Wilson, A., Svirydzenka, N., Venkateswaran, C., Kumar, M., Ram Kamal, S., Barrett, A., Dasan, C., Varma, A., & Banu, A. (2022d). Stigma and mental health problems in an Indian context: Perceptions of people with mental disorders in urban, rural, and tribal areas of Kerala. *International Journal of Social Psychiatry, 68*(2), 362–369. https://doi.org/10.1177/00207640221091187

Sacks, O. W. (2007). *Musicophilia: Tales of music and the brain.* Knopf.

Williams, M., & Zeilig, H. (2023). Broadening and deepening the understanding of agency in dementia. *Medical Humanities, 49*(1), 38–47. https://doi.org/10.1136/medhum-2022-012387.

Wood, S. (2020). Beyond Messiaen's birds: The post-verbal world of dementia. *Medical Humanities,46*(1), 73–83. https://doi.org/10.1136/medhum-2018-011616

2 Only the Lonely

The Tragic Last Years of Our Older Generation

Trini Stickle, Lorna E. Segall and Dana Nguyen Le

Introduction

The most pressing concerns for our elderly are not fear of a virus, immobility or dementia. They are isolation, loneliness and their consequential effects to individual well-being (Office of the Surgeon General, 2023). These effects on health and well-being are, according to Surgeon General Murthy, a crisis of epic proportions. We might misattribute our elderly's diminished social engagement to recent safety precautions enacted during COVID-19, but doing so would obscure the insidious and pervasive problem that aging and aging alone is for our elderly. On March 11, 2020, the World Health Organization declared COVID-19 a worldwide pandemic (World Health Organization, 2020). An entirely unknown virus was proving to be lethal for some. Without any known treatment or preventative measure, countries responded with swift and severe responses. Initially, these measures included the mandating of wearing of masks and physical, social distancing. The most stringent precaution restricted the congregation of people–in schools, in the workplace, in hospitals, and, most certainly, in residential centers. No friends or family members were allowed to visit persons residing in residential facilities in order to protect the elderly who were the most vulnerable population to the virus. Already at risk for isolation and loneliness, the precautions imposed by the pandemic for those residing in facilities quickly escalated these factors. At the time of writing this text, the world has mostly returned to pre-pandemic routines. Cases of COVID-19 are still active, but more manageable thanks to vaccines and public health initiatives empowering citizens to avoid infection. In the US, the CDC reports that "81% of COVID-19 deaths in 2020 (282,836) occurred among those aged 65 and over," and the age breakdown is startling: "Among adults aged 85 and over, 38.9% of COVID-19 deaths occurred in a nursing home or long-term care facility compared with 19.2% among adults aged 75–84 and 9.7% among those aged 65–74" (Tejada-Vera & Kramarow, 2022, p. 1). As the pandemic becomes more of our past than

DOI: 10.4324/9781003359463-3

our present, acknowledging the role it played in the following chapters is important.

Still, while these lockdowns may have generated a period of increased, visible isolation for the elderly, the problem of social isolation and loneliness long precedes the pandemic safety protocols. The prevalence of elderly loneliness and its negative health consequences also far extend beyond the US, extending across the greater global aging population (Surkalim et al., 2022). For over two decades, reports have shown that limited social interaction for our older generation exacerbates all causes of death, amplifies the effects of heart disease, and increases incidents of stroke, depression, dementia and/or mental decline (NIH, 2022; CDC, 2024). Plain and simple, we are social beings who thrive on and, perhaps for most of us, survive from human interaction. Without such interactions, the detrimental consequences are not surprising. Still, they should be alarming enough for us to seek ways to ameliorate these consequences for our loved ones, elderly under our care and our community members. Caregivers, too, are at risk for experiencing isolation, loneliness, and the resulting negative health issues whether they are providing care in facilities or are relatives, friends, or neighbors who provide informal caretaking in their personal time.

This collection of activities is our contribution aimed at diminishing social isolation and helping to ameliorate pervasive loneliness for our elderly who are aging in place, in residential centers, in prisons, and the many people who take on the role of caregiver. In this chapter, we present the health consequences of isolation and loneliness to contextualize the need for increasing our efforts to keep our elderly population physically and mentally engaged with others in ways that dignify their lives and support them aging gracefully.

Background

Nearly one million elderly live full-time in residential centers within the United States.[1] Numbers are comparable in the United Kingdom with a reported 730,000 retirement housing units across the UK and another 288,000 in centers for persons with dementia (MHA, 2022). An often forgotten about elderly population living in the United States are our incarcerated older adults. Representing the highest rate of incarceration in the world, the United States Federal prison system houses over 18,000 prisoners over the age of 55 (Federal Bureau of Prisons, 2024). Federal Bureau of Prisons data indicate that from 1991–2021 the percentage of inmates 55 and older escalated from just 3% to 15% (Prison Policy Initiative, 2023). It is estimated that 7% are living in prison with a form of dementia and 12% with cognitive impairment (Miller et al., 2023). Research in the area of incarcerated aging confirms the expected: years spent within prison accelerates the aging process, and the negative impact over time both physical and cognitive health (Prison Policy Initiative, 2023). In Brooke and colleagues' 2020 systematic review on dementia prevalence and care in the Western prison systems (i.e., US, UK, Australia, France and Sweden), three themes emerged: (1) the growing percentage of prisoners experiencing dementia or cognitive impairment; (2) the needs of prisoners living with dementia or cognitive impairment, and (3) the prevalence of prison staff and administration regarding lack of knowledge regarding dementia and cognitive impairment care. All three of these issues are key to the efforts of this collection: all persons living with dementia, regardless of where they reside, need meaningful daily care that include activities involving socialization and engagement (see also Du Toit et al., 2019, best care recommendations for incarcerated persons living with dementia, US, UK and France). Insufficient opportunities for meaningful physical and mental engagement for our elderly populations across living environments have recently become the centerpiece of health and well-being conversations.

It is the authors' intention that, through this book, we can highlight awareness of the effects of isolation on the human body and present feasible and accessible interventions that will yield enhanced social, physical and psychological outcomes for our aging population and their caregivers.

Health Consequences of Isolation and Loneliness

The National Institute on Aging defines loneliness as, "the distressing feeling of being alone or separated" and isolation as the "lack of social contacts and having few people to interact with regularly." According to these definitions, it is possible to live alone, but not feel lonely or socially isolated and, in contrast, an individual could feel lonely even in the company of others. In this section, we discuss several key health consequences of isolation and loneliness, but this is certainly not an exhaustive list. We attempt to capture the range and expanse of the health consequences within Table 2.1 in order to motivate increased activities provided by caregivers.

Negative Psychological or Emotional Stress and Health Consequences

To better illustrate the effect emotional stress has on the physical body, we have chosen to describe Takotsubo cardiomyopathy, or broken heart

Table 2.1 Health consequence of isolation and loneliness for older persons (age 55+)

Health consequence	Findings	Source(s)
Hospitalizations	Increased by 68%	Parmar et al. (2022)
Non-fatal coronary event	Increased by 29%	Health Resources & Services Administration (2019)
Fatal coronary event	Increased by 90%	Health Resources & Services Administration (2019)
Stroke	Increased by 32%	Health Resources & Services Administration (2019)
Dementia	Increased by as much as 50%	Singer (2018) Freak-Poli et al. (2022)
Premature death	Increased by 32%	Wang et al. (2023)
Suicidal ideation	Increased by 42%	Beutel et al. (2017)

Note: For a more extensive list of health consequences and companion discussion on the health effects of loneliness, see Stickle (forthcoming).

syndrome. The recent findings on Takotsubo cardiomyopathy demonstrate what poets and songwriters have known all of human existence: a person's emotional state affects one's mental and physical health. This syndrome makes it clear how morbidly negative affect can be on the human heart. Boyd and Solh (2020) present both the foundational work of Hikaru Sato, a Japanese physician and researcher, who documented the physical effects of emotional and psychological stressors on the heart and the current research findings in Takotsubo cardiomyopathy. Persons who experience great emotional stress such as the loss of a spouse or child, a natural disaster, or other devastating events may experience damage to their hearts as a result. The physical effects resulting from such stress can cause the heart to undergo a ballooning of the left ventricle. Persons experiencing this sudden change in the heart liken the symptoms to those associated with heart attacks: chest pain, shortness of breath, sweating and dizziness. These symptoms, however, are not caused by the same mechanism as heart attacks. Emotional or psychological stress causes increased levels of troponin and B-type natriuretic protein (BNP) which can block a coronary artery, which may result in "systolic heart failure" (Boyd & Solh, 2020, p. 25). The ballooning and the resulting transient ST-segment elevation can be detected through electrocardiogram (ECG). While many persons who experience such an episode recover, broken heart syndrome can, indeed, be life-threatening. While the precise connections between emotional distress and the heart remains a medical curiosity under investigation, Takotsubo cardiomyopathy demonstrates that our emotional, physical and social well-being are intricately related. While we may not understand the complete bio-physical mechanisms, heuristically, we understand that without social interaction and emotional well-being, our physical and mental health suffer.

Neuroscience research has shown us that the human brain is wired for social interaction (e.g., Kingsbury & Hong, 2020; Lebreton et al. 2012), and while we no longer question the importance that social interaction has on infants and children, particularly on the acquisition of language, we often fail to consider the neurocognitive effects that isolation and loneliness has on adults, particularly the older person who may be experiencing cognitive decline due to other causes. Düzel and colleagues (2019) present an overview of the neurostructural changes found in older persons who report feelings of pervasive loneliness and the outcomes associated with such changes. Chief among these changes is a reduction of gray matter volume within the left posterior superior temporal sulcus, one region associated with the processing of social information (Kanai et al., 2012). According to Düzel and colleagues, reduction in gray matter is linked to, among other areas of decline. increased depression symptoms (2019). Thus, a vicious cycle occurs when the brain is denied social stimuli, atrophy occurs in those areas of the brain decreasing their ability to process social stimuli which, then, decreases the ability to counter loneliness and its effects. Additional changes and reduction in size were shown to occur in the left amygdala, anterior hippocampus and adjacent entorhinal/parahippocampal cortex (Düzel et al., 2019). Unsurprisingly, these neurostructural changes are implicated in reduced emotional response, inability to control emotion and reduced memory.

Negative Effects of Social Isolation and Loneliness on Physical Fitness and Mobility

While it may seem reasonable to expect that physical frailty and problems with mobility increase social isolation and loneliness in the elderly, new research shows a reciprocal relationship between these factors. Several studies now implicate social isolation and loneliness in the decline of physical fitness and increased mobility disability of elderly persons (e.g., Tominda et al., 2024; Shankar et al., 2017; Bu et al., 2020). The relationship between isolation and the physical or mobility issues proves to be a vicious cycle. One factor–be it the physical decline or the social isolation–exacerbates the other. Tomida and colleagues (2024) found that as the elderly's social contacts and interactions dwindle, mobility disability can set in due to an absence of physical activity as persons live increasingly sedentary lives, absent of meeting with others. Likewise, elderly persons' who experience increased frailty that restricts walking, driving, or access to other transportation become isolated even more, resulting in an increased loneliness (Doi et al., 2021). Research also shows that the experiences of social isolation and loneliness also directly affect both gait and ability to complete activities of daily living (ADLs) (Shankar et al., 2017). Bu and colleagues found a 5% increase in "hazard of SR [self reported] falls relative to one point increase in loneliness independent of socio-demographic factors" (p. 4). Similarly, both duration and severity of isolation and loneliness has been shown to negatively impact physical performance across a range of abilities to include sit-to-stand time, gait, standing balance and gait-speed (Philip et al., 2020). The reciprocal relationship between physical health and mobility to social isolation and loneliness is staggering.

The data speak to the need for effective interventions that engage or keep older persons engaged within the world around them, specifically interacting with others. The data clearly show that an individual's discontent with their level of social interaction—however subjective that experience is—has detrimental consequences, physically and mentally. These devastating consequences are reason enough to identify simple, cost-effective ways to engage this population. We hope that the activities provided by the contributors will allow many moments of meaningful interactions that will contribute to the well-being of many of our elderly population, but also these activities will innervate the lives of all who are involved: young people, care partners, care providers, and, as we find in several chapters, even those who are simply observing the activities.

Conclusion

The isolating conditions that have long accompanied the aging process were magnified by COVID-19. The pandemic forced everyone to experience extended periods of isolation and loneliness that will leave long term imprints on our perspectives of life. Perhaps we may draw on this experience to deepen our insight and heighten our empathy for our fellow human beings who live within these restricted parameters constantly and use it as an accelerator to create a new, exciting culture of intergenerational engagement. To that end, the following chapters in this book aim to do just that: empower the reader to engage with the older adults in their lives in meaningful, fun and feasible ways. The following chapters provide a broad spectrum of ideas, additional resources and modifications that, we hope, make caring for our aging friends accessible, inviting and unintimidating.

Resources

1. Sherman, L. (2023). Resources and support for older adults living alone: A comprehensive guide. National Council on Aging. Advisor. www.ncoa.org/adviser/medical-alert-systems/support-for-older-adults-living-alone/#:~:text=Older%20adults%20living%20alone%20can,social%20engagement%20opportunities%2C%20and%20more.
2. National Institutes of Health: National Institutes on Aging. (2023). Social Isolation and Loneliness Outreach Toolkit. www.nia.nih.gov/ctctoolkit.

     This toolkit provides help for representatives within health care to spread the concern of social isolation and loneliness, providing informational materials for dissemination.
3. Americorp Seniors. https://americorps.gov/serve/americorps-seniors. This site connects seniors who are still able to share skills and knowledge with a variety of community settings.
4. The National Aging Resource Center for Engaging Adults. www.engagingolderadults.org/
5. SAGE Connect. Advocacy and Services for LGBTQ+ Elders. www.sageusa.org/x2-sageconnect/.
6. Friend to Friend America. https://friendtofriendamerica.org/.
7. Social Work License Map. Resources for Older Adult Experiencing Loneliness. https://socialworklicensemap.com/blog/social-isolation-resources-older-adults/.
8. Mind. www.mind.org.uk/information-support/tips-for-everyday-living/loneliness/useful-contacts/. Connects persons in the UK with resources to curb loneliness.
9. Age UK. www.ageuk.org.uk/our-impact/policy-research/loneliness-research-and-resources/. Connects persons with aging research and resources within the UK.
10. World Health Organization. Social Isolation and Loneliness. www.who.int/teams/social-determinants-of-health/demographic-change-and-healthy-ageing/social-isolation-and-loneliness.

Note

1 996,100 according to the American Health Care Association (2022).

References

American Health Care Association (2022). Facts & figures. www.ahcancal.org/Assisted-Living/Facts-and-Figures/Pages/default.aspx.

Beutel, M. E., Klein, E. M., Brähler, E., Reiner, I., Jünger, C., Michal, M., Wiltink, J., Wild, P. S., Münzel, T., Lackner, K. J., & Tibubos, A. N., (2017). Loneliness in the general population: prevalence, determinants and relations to mental health. *BMC Psychiatry*, *17*, 1–7.

Boyd, B., & Solh, T. (2020). Takotsubo cardiomyopathy: Review of broken heart syndrome. *Journal of the American Academy of Physician Assistants*, *33*(3), 24–29. https://doi.org/10.1097/01.JAA.0000654 368.35241.fc.

Brooke, J., Diaz-Gil, A., & Jackson, D. (2020). The impact of dementia in the prison setting: A systematic review. *Dementia*, *19*(5), 1509–1531.

Bu, F., Abell, J., Zaninotto, P., & Fancourt, D. (2020). A longitudinal analysis of loneliness, social isolation and falls amongst older people in England. *Scientific Reports*, *10*(1), 20064.

CDC. (2024). Health effects of social isolation and loneliness. www.cdc. gov/social-connectedness/risk-factors/.

Doi T., Tsutsumimoto K., Ishii H., Nakakubo S., Kurita S., Shimada H. (2021). Frailty and driving status associated with disability: A 24-month follow-up longitudinal study. *BMJ Open*, *11*, e042468. https://doi.org/10.1136/bmjopen-2020-042468

Du Toit, S. H. J., Withall, A., O'Loughlin, K., Ninaus, N., Lovarini, M., Snoyman, P., Butler, T., Forsyth, K., & Surr, C. A. (2019). Best care options for older prisoners with dementia: a scoping review. *International Psychogeriatrics*, *31*(8), 1081–1097.

Düzel, S., Drewelies, J., Gerstorf, D., Demuth, I., Steinhagen-Thiessen, E., Lindenberger, U., & Kühn, S. (2019). Structural brain correlates of loneliness among older adults. *Scientific Reports*, *9*(1), 13569. https:// doi.org/10.1038/s41598-019-49888-2

Federal Bureau of Prisons. (2024). Inmate age. www.bop.gov/about/statistics/statistics_inmate_age.jsp

Freak-Poli, R., Wagemaker, N., Wang, R., Lysen, T. S., Ikram, M. A., Vernooij, M. W., Dintica, C. S., Vernooij-Dassen, M., Melis, R. J., Laukka, E. J., & Fratiglioni, L. (2022). Loneliness, not social support, is associated with cognitive decline and dementia across two longitudinal population-based cohorts. *Journal of Alzheimer's Disease*, *85*(1), 295–308.

Health Resources & Services Administration. (2019). The "loneliness epidemic". www.hrsa.gov/enews/past-issues/2019/january-17/loneliness-epidemic.

Kanai, R., Bahrami, B., Duchaine, B., Janik, A., Banissy, M. J., & Rees, G. (2012). Brain structure links loneliness to social perception. *Current Biology*, *22*(20), 1975–1979.

Kingsbury, L., & Hong, W. (2020). A multi-brain framework for social interaction. *Trends in Neurosciences*, *43*(9), 651–666. https://preprints.jmir.org/preprint/28022

Lebreton, M., Barnes, A., Miettunen, J., Peltonen, L., Ridler, K., Veijola, J., . . . & Murray, G. K. (2009). The brain structural disposition to social interaction. *European Journal of Neuroscience*, *29*(11), 2247–2252.

MHA. (2022). Facts & stats about older people. www.mha.org.uk/get-involved/policy-influencing/facts-stats/.

Miller, M. C., Salgado, G., Nasrallah, N., Bronson, J., Sabatino, C. P., & Mintzer, J. (2023). Dementia in the incarcerated population: a retrospective study using the South Carolina Alzheimer's disease registry, USA. *International Journal of Prisoner Health*, *19*(1), 109–124.

National Academies of Sciences, Division of Behavioral, Social Sciences, Medicine Division, Board on Behavioral, Sensory Sciences, Board on Health Sciences Policy, Committee on the Health, Medical Dimensions of Social Isolation, and Loneliness in Older Adults (2020). *Social isolation and loneliness in older adults: Opportunities for the health care system*. National Academies Press.

NIH. (2022). Social isolation, loneliness in older people pose health risks. www.nia.nih.gov/news/social-isolation-loneliness-older-people-pose-health-risks.

Office of the Surgeon General. (2023). Our epidemic of loneliness and isolation: The U.S. Surgeon General's Advisory on the health effects of social connection and community. www.hhs.gov/sites/default/files/surgeon-general-social-connection-advisory.pdf

Parmar, M., Ma, R., Attygalle, S., Mueller, C., Stubbs, B., Stewart, R., & Perera, G. (2022). Associations between loneliness and acute hospitalisation outcomes among patients receiving mental healthcare in South London: a retrospective cohort study. *Social Psychiatry and Psychiatric Epidemiology*, *57*, 397–410. https://doi.org/10.1007/s00127-021-02079-9.

Philip, K. E., Polkey, M. I., Hopkinson, N. S., Steptoe, A., & Fancourt, D. (2020). Social isolation, loneliness and physical performance in older-adults: Fixed effects analyses of a cohort study. *Scientific Reports*, *10*(1), 13908. https://doi.org/10.1038/s41598-020-70483-3

Prison Policy Initiative. (2023). The aging prison population: Causes, costs, and consequences. www.prisonpolicy.org/blog/2023/08/02/aging/

Shankar, A., McMunn, A., Demakakos, P., Hamer, M., & Steptoe, A. (2017). Social isolation and loneliness: Prospective associations with functional status in older adults. *Health Psychology*, *36*(2), 179–209.

Singer, C. (2018). Health effects of social isolation and loneliness. *Journal of Aging Life Care*, *28*(1), 4–8.

Stickle, T. (forthcoming). Reducing the effects of loneliness in the elderly: Enacting the "principle of linguistic gratuity." In Lihe Huang & Boyd Davis (Eds.) *Language, ageing and society: What can linguistics do for the ageing world?* Palgrave.

Surkalim, D. L., Luo, M., Eres, R., Gebel, K., van Buskirk, J., Bauman, A., & Ding, D. (2022). The prevalence of loneliness across 113 countries: Systematic review and meta-analysis. *BMJ*, *376*, e067068. https://doi.org/10.1136/bmj-2021-067068

Tejada-Vera, B., & Kramarow, E. A. (2022, October). COVID-19 mortality in adults aged 65 and over: United States, 2020. CDC. NCHS Data Brief No. 446. www.cdc.gov/nchs/products/databriefs/db446.htm#print

Tomida, K., Shimoda, T., Nakajima, C., Kawakami, A., & Shimada, H. (2024). Social isolation/loneliness and mobility disability among older adults. *Current Geriatrics Reports*, 1–7. https://doi.org/10.1007/s13670-024-00414-x

Wang, F., Gao, Y., Han, Z., Yu, Y., Long, Z., Jiang, X., Wu, Y., Pei, B., Cao, Y., Ye, J., & Wang, M. (2023). A systematic review and meta-analysis of 90 cohort studies of social isolation, loneliness and mortality. *Nature Human Behaviour*, 7(8), 1307–1319.

World Health Organization. (2020). Archived: WHO timeline—COVID-19. www.who.int/news/item/27-04-2020-who-timeline-covid-19

3 Providing an Activities Menu

Goals and Chapter Preview

Lorna E. Segall and Trini Stickle

Introduction

The following chapter previews aim to briefly describe and connect the contexts in which they highlight. Each chapter features an intergenerational component highlighting meaningful methods of engaging with persons with dementia and their caregivers through a variety of creative interventions. These interventions and activities are also chosen for their feasibility and adaptability, making them appropriate for a variety of settings and resources and can utilize the strengths of the individual facilitating their implementation.

Chapter Previews

We begin with Chapter 4, which incorporates the work of William Shakespeare's final play *The Tempest* as a point of focus for learning more and creating a commonplace book. Dr. Gillian Knoll details how caregivers, in partnership with their aging family members, can create their own written products through the historical practice of commonplace books. Primarily associated with the Renaissance period, commonplace books offer a genre of writing that functions as a depository for collecting various thoughts and ideas meaningful to the reader. For example, these collections of personal artifacts may include the following: images, quotes, memories, or song lyrics identified as meaningful by the individual. These books are not intended to follow a specific format or even be a coherent collection of thoughts, which allows their creators the freedom of designing a book unique to their own interpretation and ability. Specifically for persons with dementia and their caregivers, this activity serves to honor the cognitive capabilities of the individual, offer meaningful interactions for caregivers, and highlight the creative power of reading and writing. This chapter empowers the reader to learn how to create their own commonplace book to enrich the caregiving experience.

DOI: 10.4324/9781003359463-4

Expanding on the power of writing, intergenerational engagement and creativity, Chapter 5 examines a haiku-making activity to foster self-confidence and enhance personal identity for those living with dementia. Through one-hour workshops, old and young adults alike learn about the art of haiku-making, partner to co-create their own haikus, and share their poems with other members of the workshop. To gain a deeper understanding of the experience, the authors, Dr. Yoshiko Matsumoto and her graduate assistants Harumi Maeda and Emily Wan explore the benefits of these workshops through post session interviews with the participants. Through the authors' insightful analysis and discussion of the participants' recorded verbal and non-verbal interactions, they illustrate how Haiku-making, and by extension other generative, creative activities, can benefit the aging population, our youth and caregivers. The authors provide step-by-step guidelines and resources for conducting this activity. This chapter, as with many that follow it, also demonstrates the powerful effects on well-being of intergenerational engagement.

In Chapter 6, we learn about an Artist in Residence (AIR) program which, too, features the impact of intergenerational engagement, focusing on college students living alongside residents within a personal care facility. Each academic year, author and editor Dr. Lorna Segall places two university students into a local long-term residential facility where they live for free, full-time, in exchange for intergenerational engagement, community building and friendship. Methods of creative engagement can happen through any medium which the students feel particularly empowered to offer. Authors Mackenzie Leighty, Caroline Mwenda and Kaitlyn Beard provide first-hand accounts of the benefits to students and their experiences with residents who are engaged in a variety of activities that have included art classes, singing/active music making and storytelling. To advocate for the future development of such programming, this chapter offers program development suggestions, intervention/activity ideas from the previous and current AIRs, and insight from the facility staff, administrators and resident families. So far, each of these chapters have demonstrated how poetry and creative writing support persons with dementia, community members and their caregivers.

Voices in Motion, a community choir, continues the thread of active, intergenerational engagement in Chapter 7. Founder and researcher Dr. Debra Sheets provides an overview of Voices in Motion (ViM), a professionally directed choir designed to reduce the risk of social isolation and the stigmas that are frequently attached to the dementia population through intergenerational engagement, inclusion of caregivers and community outreach concerts. For adults living with dementia, and their caregivers, the risk for depression, social isolation and caregiver distress are high. Through intergenerational engagement, the community building activity of group singing, and the final concert, persons with dementia and their caregivers can enhance their quality of life, rewrite the narrative on what it means to live with dementia, and advocate for the inclusion of this population in community settings. Furthermore, this chapter highlights not only the benefits for the individuals who participate in them, but also advocates for the feasible and cost-effective programming of community choirs. Remaining active is an important element of aging well for any population and this chapter provides the resources to begin a ViM or a similar dementia-community choir.

While the importance of remaining active can never be overstated, compliance to any exercise program can be challenging at any age. For older adults, finding methods of motivating them to engage in movement activities is paramount to aging well, but it can improve strength, balance, brain function and additional biopsychosocial benefits. In Chapter 8, we learn about the 10-week Bingocize® evidence-based wellness program from its creator Dr. K. Jason Crandall. This program offers a unique solution to physically engaging seniors by combining exercise with the familiar activity of Bingo. As research is beginning to show the incredible health benefits of this program, particularly in the reduction of falls participants experience, widespread adoption of Bingocize® is occurring within residential centers in the US and Canada, and increasingly across Europe. Bingocize® offers a flexible curriculum that addresses the specific needs of its participants and can be offered in-person or via a virtual platform, a flexibility in programming resulting from our COVID-19 precautions. Consequently, the pandemic presented an abundance of opportunities for everyone to reconsider what engagement looks like.

In another reaction to COVID-19 precautions that prevented students from meeting with persons in the residential centers, this chapter discusses the alternative ways a university student group remained engaged with the older, and most vulnerable, population. Chapter 9 presents the impact that university student organizations can have on reducing loneliness and isolation along with their negative health effects across participant ages. This chapter provides three activities along with reflections of the time spent within local residential facilities by the authors of the chapter, Dr. Trini Stickle, Prof. Jessica L. Folk and student leader Cameron Fontes. Their student organization Companions of Respected Elders (CORE) first implemented the TimeSlips© 2021 program that works to innervate the lives of elderly persons through evidenced-based, collaborative storytelling. When COVID-19 struck the United States in spring of 2020, CORE members were unable to meet with persons in residential centers due to safety precautions. In response, they began a postcard campaign that allowed persons in the residential centers to respond with the help of nursing aids and family members and which also attracted other campus participants. Lastly, the students created a writing workshop video for members of a local seniors' group. These interactions helped mitigate the consequential isolation and loneliness of aging, exasperated by the COVID-19 pandemic. Despite the unusual circumstances that engendered the later activities, the authors advocate that such interaction is needed for elderly persons in residential centers, home care and prison settings and is equally needed to create an empathetic and engaged next generation. Isolation is a primary area of concern for persons living with dementia. What can these individuals do to feel connected when their caregivers are not present? How can the dementia population remain connected, valued and heard in the absence of their caregiver or community? Relationships with our fellow human beings are crucial to our wellbeing, and evidence also suggests that our connections with our pets can provide just as meaningful of a connection.

Animatronic pets such as the Joy for All™ cats and puppies can provide empathic comfort and connection whether the person with dementia is alone or with a caregiver. Chapter 10 discusses issues that surfaced in Dr. Meredith Troutman-Jordan's special topics experiential learning/ research course, which used these pets. Student and participant experiences spilled over into videos, and workshops that addressed specific strategies for utilizing the pet (Troutman-Jordan, 2021). Dr. Troutman-Jordan, along with fellow researchers Dr. Boyd H. Davis and Dr. Margaret Maclagan, discusses the observed benefits that animatronic pets have on residents of long-term facilities. Importantly, they show how interactions with these "pets" increased language production and led to positive mood changes, noticed by caregivers and family members. The animatronic pets provided non-judgmental listeners for the care recipients, who often hesitated to talk to other people. Verbal interactions with their "pet" were often not very long or complex, but the elderly persons clearly enjoyed their robotic companions. This chapter discusses the value of a "pet" companion to ease loneliness when nobody else can be there with them. It includes several conversation starters and topics for persons living with dementia.

In Chapter 11, editors Drs. Trini Stickle and Lorna Segall synthesize the connections of Part II chapters with a forward-looking perspective on implementing health humanities as part of clinician education and caregiver workshops. To that end, they look at ways in which an interdisciplinary program could be implemented as early as undergraduate education. They conclude with a look at how such implementation and, consequently, the use of humanities-inspired activities could benefit geriatric and dementia care as well as to other patient populations.

Reference

Troutman-Jordan, M. (2021). Interdisciplinary collaboration for experiential learning in gerontology research. https://teaching.charlotte.edu/teaching-transformation/sotl-grants-program

Part II

4 Not So Commonplace

Aging, Memory and Shakespeare

Gillian Knoll

Objectives

By the end of this chapter:

1. You are expected to better understand the benefits of humanities-based activities involving Shakespeare on enhancing creativity and memory in aging populations.
2. You should be able to conduct the two activities described in this chapter using the materials and steps provided.
3. You should be able to instruct others in conducting the activities described in this chapter, and/or generate similar activities to do or share, including the optional extension activities suggested at the end of this chapter.
4. You should be able to provide a rationale for such activities based on the theoretical and empirical support provided in this chapter.

Introduction

Some of Shakespeare's most memorable lines are reflections on the aging process, from the famous description of Cleopatra as one whom "age cannot wither. . . nor custom stale her infinite variety" (*Antony and Cleopatra* 2.2.276) to Graziano's bold declaration, "with mirth and laughter, let old wrinkles come" (*The Merchant of Venice* 1.1.85). Cleopatra may be impervious to wrinkles, but Graziano anticipates them with pleasure; they are, for him, a way of remembering a full and joyful life. For many members of the elderly population, however, life experiences can be difficult to recollect and share. Activities such as scrapbooking, creating family archives and self-writing have been shown to cue memories and create positive, meaningful experiences for aging persons

DOI: 10.4324/9781003359463-6

(Allen, 2009; West et al., 2007), particularly for those with cognitive impairments (Lindley, 2012). Drawing from research on the social, emotional and cognitive benefits of such activities, I present two sequential humanities-based experiences that use Shakespeare's plays to engage elders in artful and creative processes of recollection. In these parallel activities, caregivers and their aging patients or loved ones will (1) create a commonplace book, the Renaissance equivalent of a reading journal, and (2) maintain their commonplace books as they read Shakespeare's final sole-authored play, *The Tempest* (1611).

The Tempest has been considered Shakespeare's farewell to the theater, and scholars have long speculated that Shakespeare's aging protagonist, Prospero, might have offered the playwright a chance to reflect on his own past: his career in the theater, his fame and power, his personal relationships, his failings and his blessings (Orgel, 1987). These activities give aging populations the opportunity to share in this process—both Shakespeare's and Prospero's—by recording memorable passages from the play interspersed with various artifacts such as family photos, song lyrics, news clippings, self-writing and even doodles. In this chapter, I describe in detail both activities, (1) Creating a Commonplace Book and (2) Commonplacing *The Tempest*, along with supplemental extension activities which incorporate documentary films that explore Shakespeare's significance in modern settings. In addition, I provide empirical evidence for the benefits of creating and maintaining a commonplace book to support elders as they access, curate and share their personal memories.

Context

I designed a commonplace book project for the first time in the fall of 2022 for students enrolled in Survey of British Literature I, an undergraduate English course I teach at Western Kentucky University. In some ways, the project was a response to the COVID-19 pandemic and its ripple effect on the reading community I strive to cultivate in my literature classroom. The pandemic diffused some of the energy and sociability of our dynamic classroom discussions around literature, and I was concerned that the practice of reading was becoming too solitary during an already isolating period. Historically, reading has *not* been a solitary enterprise. In Shakespeare's day (and indeed, much earlier), readers found a variety of ways to mark their lively presence in and engagement with texts, whether by jotting down notes in the margins or recording their favorite passages in a commonplace book (Mayer, 2016; Johanson, 2016; Hooks, 2012). When I introduce the art of commonplacing to my students, I describe it as an early modern version of social media—it is, at a basic level, a way of "liking" a piece of text.[1] A form of collaborative reading, commonplacing has offered readers ways of talking back to their texts, of capturing their emotional reactions, and of making creative connections with others. For my students returning to the classroom after lockdown, maintaining commonplace books helped them organize and share their reading experiences with fellow classmates. At the beginning of each week, students gathered in pairs or small groups to discuss their favorite commonplace book entries, and at the end of the term, they presented the finished products to the class.

The success of this project (which I have adapted for other literature classes, including a course on Shakespeare) inspired the activities I describe in this chapter. The goal is for elders and caregivers to engage meaningfully with a Shakespeare play while making broader connections, activating personal memories and making art. In Shakespeare's day, commonplace books were considered an "indispensable tool for the Renaissance reader" (Hooks, 2012), but they are infinitely adaptable in the present moment. A *New York Times* "Tech Tip" from 2021 describes them as "somewhat like marking your favorite lines in a novel with the Amazon Kindle highlights[2] feature—except your personal one-stop knowledge repository can also include song lyrics, movie dialogue, poems, recipes, podcast transcripts, and any inspiring bits you find in your reading and listening" (Biersdorfer, 2021). Many of my students chose to create a digital commonplace book where they interspersed memorable quotations from early British literature with contemporary memes, links to YouTube videos, news articles, or favorite lines from novels, pop songs, films and television shows. Others opted to handwrite in a blank book, copying quotations from premodern literary texts alongside their own doodles, magazine clippings, or personal artifacts. Figure 4.1 features an image of a commonplace book created by a student in my Shakespeare class in the spring of 2023.

Following in her family's tradition of scrapbooking, Kate arranged materials that reflected her abiding interests in fashion, art and international travel alongside handwritten quotations from Shakespeare's *Antony and Cleopatra*. This commonplace book was artful and meaningful; its display of text and image reflected broader connections between past and present, word and action, imagination and memory.

Such connections are particularly significant for members of aging populations, especially those who struggle with memory—persons with difficulty retrieving and sharing personal memories, as well as those who struggle with short-term recall. As Renaissance scholar Desidarus Erasmus wrote in his famed humanist treatise *De Copia* (1512), commonplace books can help a reader to "fix what you have read more firmly in your mind" (Brayman Hackel, 2005, p. 146). Sometimes this process of "fix[ing]. . . in your mind" requires little more than copying out a passage by hand; sometimes it asks us to arrange or contextualize a piece of text. While some commonplace books are indexed and organized into

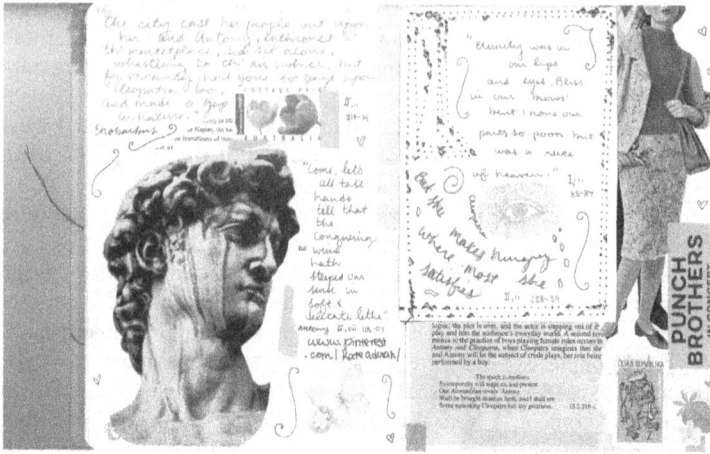

Figure 4.1 Commonplace book entries on Shakespeare's *Antony and Cleopatra* by Kate Fisher, student

Source: Matt Bryant

categories, others might be generically incoherent; there is no need for a prevailing logic or sequence that governs its pages. As elderly participants weave together memorable passages from Shakespeare with personal artifacts, they might form new connections and reconstruct their own histories artfully alongside Shakespeare's language. Research in the social sciences has demonstrated that "memories are not retrieved but are formed; narratives are actively reconstructed (and co-constructed with others); a life story is interpreted and retrospectively reinterpreted" (Lindley, 2012, p. 15). By interspersing Shakespeare's language with materials that are personally meaningful to readers, this project honors the power of reading and writing to shape memories and make them new.

Creating a Commonplace Book: Activity 1 Summary

The goal of this activity is to create a reading journal that can be used to record memorable quotations from Shakespeare's *The Tempest*, which is the focus of Activity 2. Because commonplace books can take a variety of forms, this activity is quite flexible and easily adjustable to meet the needs and interests of elderly participants. For those participants who are artistically inclined, the commonplace book might be a kind of scrapbook arranged in a graphic style, with text from Shakespeare supplementing images of various sorts. For those who are interested in preserving personal or family memories, commonplace books can take the form of an album, with quotations from Shakespeare placed alongside artifacts from one's life. And those who prefer to maintain a more traditional commonplace book can focus on assembling memorable passages from Shakespeare (and elsewhere), perhaps organizing them into categories that are personally significant or useful. Participants are also free to choose how much of their own history—and how much of Shakespeare's language—to include in their commonplace books. Those with deficits in memory retrieval may find it easiest to decenter personal or family artifacts and instead to focus on collecting quotations from Shakespeare's play (perhaps also from other reading material, from media like television or films, from casual conversations, etc.) or on illustrating Shakespeare's text with drawings or collages.

Caregivers will begin the activity by sharing images of commonplace books (many of them housed in museums and research libraries around the world—some elaborate and artful, others plainer and functional) to learn about their historical uses. Readers in Shakespeare's day copied their favorite passages from poetry or songs into their commonplace books (Johanson, 2016; Estill, 2015), but they also added illustrations, recipes, jokes, lists of domestic items, diary entries, notes to loved ones, and their own pieces of creative writing (Brayman Hackel, 2005). In the centuries that followed, writers such as Lewis Carroll, Virginia Woolf and Mark Twain kept commonplace books, often to preserve memorable turns of phrase for later use. Examples from these commonplace books and others can be found on websites such as thecommonplacebookproject.com. After exploring examples, each participant will select a format for their own commonplace book. Once they set up their commonplace book and create a title page, they are ready to move on to Activity 2, Commonplacing *The Tempest*. I present a generic set of materials and steps to follow for Activity 1, but caregivers should feel free to make adjustments based on interactions with participants.

Materials

1. A notebook (e.g., blank book, spiral notebook, composition book, notepad, journal) for each elderly participant.
2. Writing implement(s).
3. Basic art supplies like scissors, tape/glue sticks and assorted markers/colored pencils.
4. A computer, tablet, or printouts to explore commonplace book examples linked in the *New York Times* (Biersdorfer, 2021). For specific examples, see linked images of commonplace books by John Milton, John Locke and Sir Alec Guinness.

5. Personal artifacts (e.g., family photos, postcards, letters, ticket stubs, invitations/thank-you cards, artwork from grandchildren, news clippings) and/or a diverse stack of magazines/newspapers for clippings.

Steps to Activity

1. Participants and caregivers meet in a space that includes a comfortable work surface, ideally a large table where supplies can be spread out.
2. To begin the activity, caregivers introduce the concept of a commonplace book, including its historical context, and share images of commonplace books for inspiration.
3. Participants choose a basic format for their commonplace books. If in a group setting, participants can brainstorm ideas with others in small groups or pairs.
4. With assistance from caregivers, participants organize their commonplace books with a title page and, if desired, a table of contents or index to list possible categories (e.g., friendship, family, humor). For suggestions on categories and formats, see Biersdorfer (2021).
5. To conclude the activity, participants discuss ideas for arranging Shakespeare quotes alongside other materials, whether personal artifacts, magazine clippings, other illustrations, or short forms of self-writing.

Reflection

Research in the field of creative aging has demonstrated the numerous and significant benefits of hands-on arts activities such as scrapbooking on the physical health, mental health, functionality, and overall well-being of older persons (National Endowment of the Arts, 2006; Boyer, 2007). Creating a Commonplace Book is essentially a craft project—an opportunity for participants to express themselves creatively and to work with their hands—with a foundation in the humanities. Participants with interests in art or artmaking can focus on creating a decorative cover and title page for their commonplace book. Alternatively, if participants are more interested in literary or book history, it may be helpful to devote extra time to reviewing examples from historically significant writers and thinkers before setting up their own commonplace books. Participants might also reflect on and discuss their own reading and writing practices alongside those of various historical models. The main tasks of the caregiver in this activity are (1) to present options, (2) to engage participants in conversations about commonplace books (historical examples and their own), (3) to provide or procure materials, and (4) to follow the lead of the participant, attending to their unique interests, abilities, needs and wishes. At the conclusion of this activity, it will be helpful to assure participants that they can make changes to their commonplace books at any time, particularly if they discover a more appropriate format once they begin reading Shakespeare's play. From this point, participants are ready to proceed to Activity 2, Commonplacing *The Tempest*.

Commonplacing *The Tempest*: Activity 2 summary

This activity draws from a long tradition of excerpting Shakespeare's language and recording it in a commonplace book for future contemplation or study. Scholars of early modern literature and culture have traced this practice to Shakespeare's own lifetime, as early as 1600, observing that "commonplaces from Shakespeare's works were part of quotidian seventeenth-century life, found in schools, churches, and conversations" (Estill, 2015, p. 149). The goal of this activity is to promote an active reading experience of *The Tempest* with elders by forging intellectual, aesthetic and personal connections with Shakespeare's language. Activity 2 takes place over the course of five meetings that occur at regular intervals; simplest would be a schedule of one 60–90-minute meeting per week over a five-week period. Each meeting will focus on one act of *The Tempest* (there are five acts in all), with two main objectives: first, to discuss one act of the play with caregivers (and each other, if the activity is conducted in a group setting), and second, to maintain and share commonplace books. Some participants may prefer to add entries to their commonplace books while reading each act of *The Tempest* on their own, some might wait until meetings to update their commonplace books, and others might develop a routine that incorporates both of these practices. (For example, participants might mark passages in their books but wait to copy them out until meeting with caregivers. Or they might record the quotations but wait until the meetings to adorn their commonplace book entries with supplementary artifacts or images.)

Each commonplace meeting proceeds in three basic stages. First, participants share with caregivers (and each other, if in a group setting) passages or episodes from *The Tempest* they have noted during the week, including questions about Shakespeare's plot, character, or language. Second, caregivers facilitate a brief discussion of the play. Third, participants and caregivers work collaboratively on commonplace books.

The first and third stages of each meeting are fairly straightforward—steps are outlined later in this section—but because the discussion of *The Tempest* may feel more challenging for caregivers to facilitate, I offer additional support here. Specifically, I suggest that caregivers identify a few key themes from *The Tempest* that are introduced in the play's opening act. Participants are welcome to organize their commonplace book according to those categories, along with any others that interest them. The following four themes can scaffold each discussion of the play: (1) memory, (2) power, (3) relationships (family/friendship), and (4) imagination.[3] Depending on participant interest, certain themes might be discussed in greater depth during a particular meeting, but all four can be traced throughout Shakespeare's play.

The Tempest is Shakespeare's final sole-authored play, a comedy about an aging duke, Prospero, who has been stranded on an island with his daughter for twelve years after his brother conspired to overthrow him. Prospero is an accomplished magician, and after twelve years of dedicated study, he decides to use his power (along with a good deal of luck, conniving and political savvy) to bring his enemies to the island and, he hopes, to justice. *The Tempest* has all the makings of a tragedy: it features a single protagonist, a powerful person of noble birth, who seeks vengeance and inflicts a good deal of harm on others. But although Prospero is a shadowy and complex character, he chooses forgiveness in the end. The play's comic ending includes scenes of reconciliation, anticipation and remembering. For Prospero, looking back is essential to the process of moving forward.

Caregivers and participants might read a basic summary of *The Tempest* before beginning the play, and/or they might read aloud the preceding paragraph to become acquainted with the basic plot of the play. At the first meeting about Act 1, caregivers can identify the four themes listed above and solicit feedback from participants about how each theme is established in the play's opening act, which is comprised of two extremely dissonant scenes. The first scene, which stages a shipwreck of Prospero's enemies, is short, action packed and present tense. The second scene, in which Prospero unfolds to his daughter Miranda their family's history, is much lengthier, more expository and backward looking, a reflection of the play's "profoundly retrospective quality," as scholar Stephen Orgel puts it in his introduction to the play. Orgel has observed that *The Tempest* "is deeply involved in recounting and re-enacting past action, in evoking and educating the memory" (1987, p. 5). Early conversations with participants might focus on the role of recollection in Prospero's self-concept and in his relationships with others, what scholar Evelyn Tribble has called "the intersubjective nature of memory" (2006, p. 155). Participants might collect quotations that reveal Prospero's struggle with this intersubjectivity in his expository speeches. (For example, he repeatedly interrupts his reminiscences in Act 1 to make sure his daughter is paying attention.) They might also find it helpful to compare their own processes of remembering with Prospero's, especially as they collaborate with caregivers (and possibly one another) to recall passages from the play and display them in commonplace books each week.

Below I present a list of materials and steps to follow for Activity 2. I have included supplementary materials/optional steps to provide increased flexibility. For additional support in finding quotations from Shakespeare's play that are well suited to this activity, please see the appendix to this chapter, which lists a few key passages from *The Tempest* about memory.

Materials

1. Commonplace books and all the materials listed in Activity 1.
2. A modern edition of Shakespeare's *The Tempest* that includes editorial glosses. (I recommend the Folger Shakespeare Library edition, which includes a short summary of each scene and helpful editorial glosses on each facing page. See Resources at the end of this chapter for more information.)

Optional: A modern filmed production of *The Tempest* to supplement reading. Most widely accessible is the 2010 film directed by Julie Taymor, starring Helen Mirren as "Prospera" (a female version of Shakespeare's Prospero). See References for bibliographic information.

Steps to Activity

1. Participants take approximately a week to read one act of Shakespeare's *The Tempest* independently. (If desired, and if resources are available, participants might watch parts of a modern filmed production.)
2. Participants and caregivers meet in a space that includes a comfortable work surface—ideally, a large table where supplies can be spread out.
3. In the first part of the meeting, participants will be invited to share memorable passages from their reading of the play.

4. In the second part of the meeting, participants and caregivers will discuss the play. Discussions can be freeform or can be scaffolded according to the categories listed in the preceding section.
5. The third part of the meeting is devoted to collaborative work on commonplace books. Participants and caregivers can use this time to (1) record memorable passages, (2) organize passages into groupings or categories, (3) add illustrations or other visual materials, and/or (4) include additional text, perhaps quotations from other sources or any form of self-writing.
6. Subsequent meetings will follow this basic format. I suggest scheduling one meeting for each act of Shakespeare's five-act comedy. Caregivers might extend the length of the first and final meetings to provide extra time for discussions of the play.

Reflection

Along with passages from *The Tempest,* other materials (e.g., illustrations, quotations from other sources) can be added and arranged with the help of caregivers during meetings. Caregivers and participants can return to the historical models from Activity 1 for inspiration at any time, and I have included additional examples from my student (see Figures 4.2 and 4.3) to showcase the range of approaches one might take. In Figure 4.2, quotations from *A Midsummer Night's Dream* are handwritten on a variety of materials: a postcard, magazine clippings, a scrap of paper. Participants who adopt a similar practice might keep an archive of personal artifacts, clippings, or scraps of paper nearby as they read the play, selecting their writing materials based on the language in their quote (e.g., a passage about the setting might be scribbled on a postcard or ticket stub). These participants might wait until meeting with caregivers before arranging their collection of quotations within their commonplace books.

Figure 4.3 illustrates additional possibilities for personalizing one's commonplace book. Kate's entries on *Henry V* included a travel souvenir and a quotation that featured her own name (Princess Katherine, or "Kate," as Henry calls her, is a character in Shakespeare's play). These choices enabled Kate to capture and reflect on language from the play that might not hold as much significance for someone else but were meaningful to her. Not all quotations are personal; some are chosen for their style, some their sounds, some for a more generic message. As there is no need to contextualize or justify passages copied into commonplace books, participants should feel free to select quotations for any number of reasons and arrange them as they see fit.

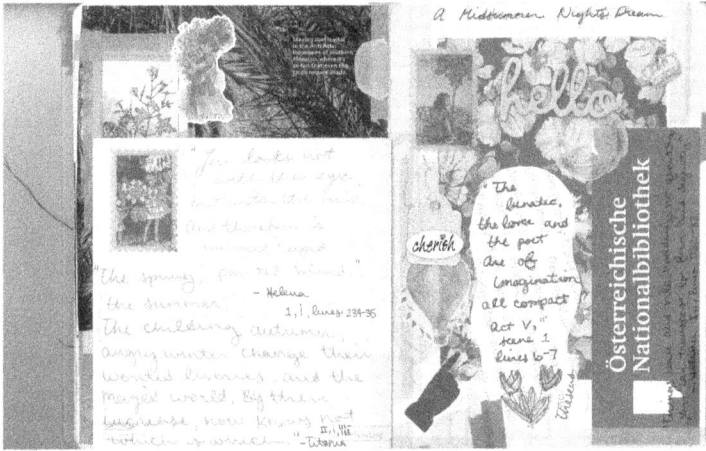

Figure 4.2 Commonplace book entries on Shakespeare's *A Midsummer Night's Dream,* by student Kate Fisher

Source: Matt Bryant

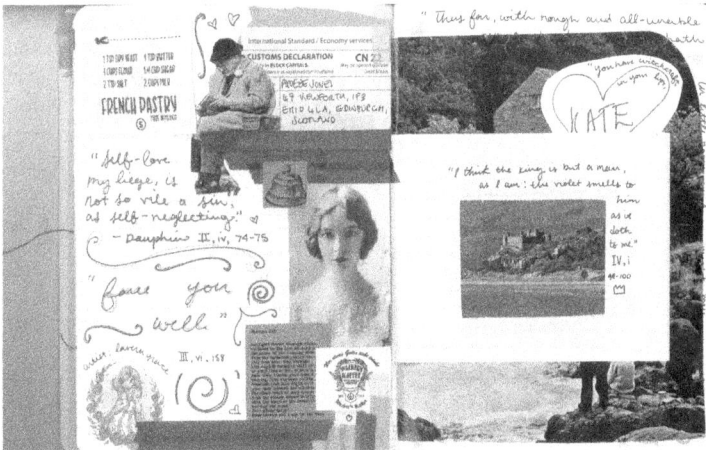

Figure 4.3 Commonplace book entries on Shakespeare's *Henry V,* by student Kate Fisher

Source: Matt Bryant

Optional Supplementary Activities: Commonplacing Shakespeare on the Screen

After completing the above activities, elders may be interested in (1) adding entries to their commonplace books and/or (2) exploring Shakespeare's language in new contexts. One option for pursuing these interests is to extend the commonplacing practices developed in Activity 2 to documentary films that explore Shakespeare's plays in modern settings. Two accessible films that would pair exceptionally well with the above activities are *Shakespeare Behind Bars* (2005) and *Still Dreaming* (2014), both directed by Hank Rogerson and produced by Jilann Spitzmiller. The award-winning documentary *Shakespeare Behind Bars* follows a group of inmates from Luther Luckett Correctional Facility in LaGrange, Kentucky, as they rehearse and perform *The Tempest*. The inmates make powerful connections between the play and their own lives—their relationships, their crimes, their feelings about the past, their hopes for the future—as they inhabit Shakespeare's characters. For elderly participants who have just read *The Tempest* and have perhaps made similar connections, the documentary film has much to offer; quotations from the film would not only enrich their commonplace books but also their conversations about Shakespeare's significance in the present day. The production team behind *Shakespeare Behind Bars* released another documentary film that is uniquely relevant to our aging populations, as it takes place in an assisted-living facility. *Still Dreaming*, a similarly retrospective film, follows a group of residents from Lillian Booth Actors Home in Englewood, New Jersey, many of whom are retired entertainers, as they rehearse and eventually perform Shakespeare's *A Midsummer Night's Dream*. Viewing, discussing and commonplacing this film presents opportunities for elders to reflect on their own relationship to the arts and creativity. They might also consider the capacity of Shakespeare's language to give voice to their own experiences and their unique talents and challenges as aging individuals.

Below I present a list of materials and basic steps to follow for these supplementary activities. For either or both films, caregivers should feel free to add extra meetings to continue work on commonplace books (and to share them with others), as time and resources allow.

Materials

1. Commonplace books and all the materials listed in Activity 1.
2. Equipment and space for screening films (computer/projector or a large television, and a gathering space or meeting room with comfortable seating).

3. One or both of the following documentary films: (1) *Shakespeare Behind Bars* (Rogerson, 2005), which has streaming and DVD options available online at shakespearebehindbars.org/ documentary; (2) *Still Dreaming* (Rogerson and Spitzmiller, 2014), with streaming and DVD options available online at stilldreamingmovie.com. Jilann Spitzmiller has made *Still Dreaming* available for free streaming at https://vimeo.com/ 263786714.

Steps to Activity

1. Participants and caregivers gather in a space that is equipped for screening a film. Participants bring their commonplace books (or, if preferred, a notepad or other writing materials) and writing implements.
2. Caregivers briefly introduce the film before screening it in its entirety. Introductions are available on each film's website: shakespearebehindbars.org/documentary and StillDreaming-Movie.com.
3. After the film concludes, caregivers invite participants to discuss memorable moments of the film. Participants are welcome to record any thoughts or quotes from the film in their commonplace books during this conversation.
4. A second meeting takes place soon after the screening in which participants and caregivers add materials from the film to their commonplace books. Ideally the film is still accessible for any participants who would like to review a scene.

Optional: Repeat the above steps for the second documentary film.

Optional: Add extra meetings to extend conversations and work on commonplace books, if desired.

Reflection

After *Still Dreaming* was released in 2014, the filmmakers generated a robust body of supplemental materials, such as behind-the-scenes interviews and discussion questions. Caregivers are encouraged to consult the *Still Dreaming* Discussion Resource & Guide (Spitzmiller, 2015), available for free download at www.stilldreamingmovie.com, for support with initiating conversations about the film. Along with the discussion questions for viewers and participants, the Discussion Resource & Guide features a set of questions for caregivers and staff that can be used to prompt their discussions about planning, facilitating, or extending creative arts programs for elders. Caregivers might also consult the Guide's list of online resources for creative aging research and programs (Spitzmiller, 2015, p. 13). Perhaps the most comprehensive resource on this list is "Creativity Matters: Arts and Aging Toolkit" (Boyer, 2017), which includes helpful context for creative aging programs, an introduction to the aging services field, program design and implementation, model programs, a glossary and additional resources.

As participants add entries to commonplace books based on their responses to the films, caregivers should encourage them to experiment with multiple formats. Quotations from the films are always welcome, but elders should not feel pressured to scribble down lines from the film while they are viewing, or to recall specific turns of phrase after finishing the film. Participants might simply jot down thoughts about a particular moment or about a connection with their own life. They might write a response to one or more of the questions from the Discussion Resource & Guide in their commonplace books. Or, if they prefer to add visual rather than textual entries, they can add images, drawings, or other collage materials inspired by different scenes in the films.

Conclusion

When Shakespeare's Prospero shares memories with his daughter Miranda, he refers to their past as "the dark backward and abysm of time" (*The Tempest*, 1.2.62). While some memories are shrouded in the darkness of the past, others can live fresh in our minds through cultivation, collaboration and creativity. These activities for aging populations begin from the premise that the process of recollection can be enriched by (1) the creative arts and (2) the presence of others who are grappling with their past—whether by letting go, holding tight, moving on, or, quite simply, remembering. The characters in Shakespeare's *The Tempest* model the experience of recollection in all its messiness, complexity and intersubjectivity. Together, Shakespeare's characters create what cognitive scientist Eviatar Zerubavel has called a "remembrance environment," in which memories are both individual and social (Zerubavel, 1997). The commonplace book activities described in this chapter provide just such an environment, where elders might recall moments from their own lives, or they might make other connections prompted by Shakespeare's plays.

Since the Victorian era, readers have found in Shakespeare's language a way of shaping their own experiences, emotions, beliefs and thoughts.

Scholar Kristine Johanson calls this phenomenon "self-help Shakespeare." Commonplace books, writes Johanson, might be considered the "origins" of modern self-help books (2016, p. 1724). People look to Shakespeare for answers all the time; they have found in his language moral instruction, parental guidance, business tips, models for political leadership, ideas for spicing up their love lives, and much more. For members of our aging population, Shakespeare's words might offer what Theseus calls "a local habitation and a name" (*A Midsummer Night's Dream*, 5.1.18), a poetic way of shaping a life of rich and varied experiences. Commonplace books are just such a "local habitation," a place to hold memories from Shakespeare and from other aspects of life.

Questions to Consider

1. Which aspects of the above activities do you expect to be most rewarding for elders? What steps can you take to ensure that elders get the most out of them?
2. Which aspects of the above activities might pose the most challenges, either in planning or in execution? What steps can you take to pre-empt or mitigate those challenges?
3. How might you present any of the above activities to program administrators or funding sources to secure their support?
4. How would you structure commonplace book meetings? Where might you diverge from the suggestions provided for Activities 1 and 2?
5. To further extend the activities described in this chapter, what kinds of sources (films, books, songs, news sources, etc.) might pair well with Shakespeare excerpts in commonplace books?

Resources

1. *The Commonplace Book Project: An Informal and Scholarly Resource for Writing, Teaching, Collecting, and Studying Commonplace Books* (thecommonplacebookproject.com)
2. *The Tempest*, by William Shakespeare, Folger Shakespeare Library edition (2004). Available for purchase on Amazon (www.amazon.com/Tempest-Folger-Shakespeare-Library/dp/0743482832) and other online retailers
3. National Center for Creative Aging

4. *Creativity Matters: The Arts and Aging Toolkit* (nationalguild. org/resources/resources/free-guild-resource/creativity-matters-the-arts-and-aging-toolkit)
5. *Arts & Aging.* (www.StillDreamingMovie.com/arts-aging)

Notes

1 Rather than a thumbs up, the social media equivalent of a "like," early modern readers often drew a "manicule"—an index finger pointed sideways (see Hooks, 2012, for examples).
2 See www.amazon.com/b/?node=11627044011.
3 This is by no means an exhaustive list. Additional possibilities include nature, gender/sexuality, race, imperialism, justice, reconciliation, magic, love, books and much more.

References

Allen, R. S. (2009). The legacy project intervention to enhance meaningful family interactions: Case examples. *Clinical Gerontologist, 32*(2), 164–176. https://doi.org/10.1080/07317110802677005

Biersdorfer, J. D. (2021, February 10). Create a digital commonplace book. *New York Times.* www.nytimes.com/2021/02/10/technology/personaltech/make-digital-commonplace-book.html

Boyer, J. M. (2007). *Creativity matters: The arts and aging toolkit.* National Guild of Community Schools of the Arts. https://national-guild.org/files/resources/public/creativity-matters-the-arts-and-aging-toolkit.pdf

Brayman Hackel, H. (2005). *Reading material in early modern England: Print, gender, and literacy.* Cambridge University Press.

Estill, L. (2015). Commonplacing readers. In M. J. Kidnie & S. Massai (Eds.), *Shakespeare and textual studies* (pp. 149–162). Cambridge University Press.

Hooks, A. (2012, August). How to read like a Renaissance reader. *Anchora.* www.adamghooks.net/2012/08/how-to-read-like-renaissance-reader.html

Johanson, K. (2016). Self-help Shakespeare. In B. Smith (Ed.), *The Cambridge guide to the worlds of Shakespeare*, vol. 2 (pp. 1724–728). Cambridge University Press.

Lindley, S. E. (2012). Before I forget: From personal memory to family history. *Human–Computer Interaction, 37*, 13–36. https://doi.org/10.1080/07370024.2012.656065

Mayer, J. (2016). Reading practices. In B. Smith (Ed.), *The Cambridge guide to the worlds of Shakespeare*, vol. 1 (pp. 354–360). Cambridge University Press.

National Endowment of the Arts. (2006). *Executive summary: The impact of professionally conducted cultural programs on older adults.* The Center on Aging, Health & Humanities, The George Washington University. www.arts.gov/sites/default/files/NEA-Creativity-and-Aging-Cohen-study.pdf

Orgel, S. (1987). Introduction. In *The Tempest* (pp. 1–39). Oxford University Press.

Rogerson, H. (Director). (2005). *Shakespeare Behind Bars* [Film]. Philomath Films.

Rogerson, H., & Spitzmiller, J. (Directors). (2014). *Still dreaming* [Film]. Philomath Films.

Spitzmiller, J. (2015). *Still Dreaming* resource & discussion guide. https://stilldreamingmovie.com/stilldreamingdiscussionguideprint order9-15

Taymor, J. (Director). (2010). *The Tempest* [Film]. Touchstone Pictures; Miramax Films.

Tribble, E. B. (2006). "The Dark Backward and Abysm of Time": *The Tempest* and memory. *College Literature, 33*(1), 151–168. https://doi.org/10.1353/lit.2006.0013

West, D., Quigley, A., & Kay, J. (2007). MEMENTO: A digital-physical scrapbook for memory sharing. *Personal and Ubiquitous Computing, 11*, 313–328. https://doi.org/10.1007/s00779-006-0090-7

Zerubavel, E. (1997). *Social mindscapes: An invitation to cognitive sociology.* Harvard University Press.

Appendix

Key Passages from *The Tempest* about Memory

1.   What seest thou else
   In the dark backward and abysm of time?
                   —Prospero (1.2.61–62)

2.   by telling of it,
   Made such a sinner of his memory,
   To credit his own lie
                   —Prospero (1.2.121–22)

3.   The isle is full of noises,
   Sounds and sweet airs, that give delight and hurt not.
   Sometimes a thousand twangling instruments
   Will hum about mine ears, and sometime voices
   That, if I then had waked after long sleep,
   Will make me sleep again: and then, in dreaming,
   The clouds methought would open and show riches
   Ready to drop upon me that, when I waked,
   I cried to dream again.
                   —Caliban (3.2.148–56)

4.   Our revels now are ended. These our actors,
     As I foretold you, were all spirits and
     Are melted into air, into thin air:
     And, like the baseless fabric of this vision,
     The cloud-capp'd towers, the gorgeous palaces,
     The solemn temples, the great globe itself,
     Ye all which it inherit, shall dissolve

And, like this insubstantial pageant faded,
Leave not a rack behind. We are such stuff
As dreams are made on, and our little life
Is rounded with a sleep.
                    —Prospero (4.1.165–80)

5.   Let us not burthen our remembrances with
     A heaviness that's gone.
                    —Prospero (5.1.236–37)

6.   Now I want
     Spirits to enforce, art to enchant,
     And my ending is despair,
     Unless I be relieved by prayer
     Which pierces so that it assaults
     Mercy itself and frees all faults.
     As you from crimes would pardon'd be,
     Let your indulgence set me free.
                    —Prospero (Epilogue, 13–20)

5 On an Equal Footing

Intergenerational Haiku-Making Activity

Yoshiko Matsumoto, Harumi Maeda and Emily Wan

Objectives

By the end of this chapter:

1. You are expected to better understand the effect of the inter-generational haiku-making activity designed to encourage artistic and social interaction between older adults living with mild cognitive impairment (MCI) and younger adults through the means of haiku appreciation and creation.
2. You should be able to conduct the activity online or in-person using the materials and steps provided.
3. You should be able to instruct others in conducting the activity and/or develop similar activities.
4. You should be able to provide a rationale for such activities based on the theoretical and empirical support provided in this chapter.

Introduction

This chapter will describe an intergenerational activity of creating and appreciating haiku, a 17-syllable poetic form originating in Japan. Many residential and day services programs for older adults offer thoughtful humanities-based activities such as storytelling and creating memory books, often recruiting young volunteers to assist and collaborate with the older adults. Through engaging in such intergenerational activities, both younger and older persons gain meaningful experiences in addition to the tangible artistic products.

The haiku-making activity is designed to achieve similar goals. However, it differs from other more commonly found programs in that older and younger persons participate in the activity on an equal footing and

DOI: 10.4324/9781003359463-7

engage in the same activity independently and collaboratively. In the haiku-making activity, younger persons are not recruited for the purpose of assisting older participants to compose haiku. Instead, they also learn about haiku and create their own poems alongside the older participants. Although the participants may notice the age difference, they are all positioned simply as persons participating in the activity and are free to assist or not assist others. In a small group setting, all parties create their own haiku independently and collaboratively based on seasonal photographs of their choosing and have conversations about their haiku that may sometimes extend to stories of their personal backgrounds. The design of communal engagement in haiku creates a shared occasion that is aimed at combating loneliness by providing a chance for both older and younger persons to meet with new people and to jointly undertake an activity as fellow (and equal) participants. It is also hoped that the participants can maintain and enhance their verbal creativity, as well as experiment with and experience how good conversations can be had with persons in different life stages.

The activity can be conducted in any small intergenerational group, but we have focused on populations known to experience acute loneliness: older persons living with cognitive impairment and younger persons (Beam & Kim, 2020; Christiansen et al., 2021; see also Chapter 9). The online and in-person sessions can be formatted as a one-off session as detailed in the following section, or as a three-day session (one meeting per week for three weeks) which divides the activity into (1) an introduction to haiku (steps 1–8), (2) composing one's own haiku and a conversation between a pair of older and younger participants (steps 9–10), and (3) a whole group session for talking about one another's haiku (steps 11–13). The format of a three-day session presents an opportunity for older adults living with cognitive impairments and younger adults (undergraduate and graduate students) to benefit from more sustained and intimate social and artistic interactions through the Japanese verbal art form.

Background

The intergenerational haiku-making activity is part of the research project "Sharing Conversations: A core human experience across life" supported by a Cultivating Humanities Grant of the Changing Human Experience Initiative (School of Humanities and Sciences, Stanford University) awarded to Yoshiko Matsumoto in March 2020. The project aimed to counter a common perception that the conversation of older adults is often filled with painful self-disclosure and that people with dementia display a serious communication breakdown. Actual conversations among older adults about painful events reveal their resilience and the continuity of stable and quotidian self (e.g., Matsumoto, 2011, 2019), and discourse studies of persons living with dementia reveal that they hold conversations cooperatively with their partners, similarly to those without dementia (e.g., Hamilton, 1994, 2019; Ramanathan, 1997). A study of interaction among memory care residents and with care workers also indicated that there is rich communication, especially when the content is interpersonal and affect-related (Matsumoto, 2019), suggesting that communication breakdown is more likely experienced by those not living with dementia rather than by the residents or the care workers. The project was intended to advocate the sharing of conversations to enhance an inclusive community by illustrating the fundamental importance of interpersonal and affective interaction in language use and human communication throughout one's lifespan. To do so, the project employed detailed linguistic and narrative analyses of naturally occurring recorded conversations of older adults living with or without dementia in Japan and in the US.

The unexpected COVID-19 pandemic necessitated the original in-person-based research plan to be modified, and as a result, the online (Zoom®) haiku activity was conceived in autumn 2020. It aimed to mitigate the seriousness of social isolation, which negatively impacts all but particularly exacerbates the health conditions of cognitively impaired older adults. The idea was to offer older adults living with MCI a chance to engage in positive social interactions with younger participants and enjoy a new artistic activity together in a small non-threatening group setting, in order to help them maintain their communicative ability and creativity through verbal art. The activity was first put into practice in collaboration with a few local organizations and through personal networks in November 2020. Since then, the sessions have been sustained and later expanded in collaboration with a community partner through a Seed Grant from the Office of Community Engagement (Stanford University) to Matsumoto[1] through January–August 2023. Matsumoto's co-authors of this chapter, Harumi Maeda and Emily Wan, are core research assistants of the project[2] who substantially contributed to designing the materials and facilitating the activity sessions, as well as to the analysis of the research findings. Several other Stanford students have also been engaged in the project as research assistants or as activity participants. The sessions have been offered in person too when possible.

Haiku was chosen as the platform of the activity for several reasons. First, with its simple format of 5–7–5 syllables/morae, haiku is accessible to many people, as one can usually learn the basics and compose within a limited amount of time. Second, neither young nor older adults in the US are very familiar with this traditional Japanese poetry, if at all. Even if they have a brief prior exposure to haiku (e.g., one class in elementary school), a haiku activity presents a relatively new experience to both groups of participants. Third, while younger participants' ability to compose logically sequenced sentences may exceed that of older participants living with MCI, such complexity or logical continuity is not favored in haiku as it is in prose, and older adults with a wealth of life experience may be more attuned to express a depth of emotion. This has the effect of placing both groups on a level playing field. Fourth, following the tradition of seasonal scenes serving as topics for haiku, participants are asked to make their haiku based on a seasonal photograph they have chosen. This has two benefits: the participants have some emotional connection to the material for haiku-making so that it can elicit personal and memorable feelings, prompting deeper self-expression through the poem; and, the photograph is "physical objects in the here-and-now" (Hamilton, 2019, p. 161) which does not require recollection of specific past events, so that everyone including participants who may have memory difficulties can feel at ease.

The intergenerational haiku activity focuses on the well-being of an often "othered" and ignored population while encouraging an inclusive mindset among the young participants to foster healthy and collaborative communities. Pinkert et al. (2021) find that "the exclusions experienced by PwD [people with dementia] are social barriers that are related more to the *social relationships* [emphasis added] between people with and without dementia than to the cognitive effects of dementia" (p. 21). Further, narrative and conversational studies of persons living with dementia (Davis, 2005; Guendouzi & Müller, 2006; Hamilton, 1994; Ramanathan, 1997; Ryan et al., 2005; to name a few) illustrate the significance of verbal and nonverbal interactions as they affect the quality of communication for persons living with dementia and the maintenance of their personhood (Kitwood, 1997).

Through the haiku activity, we explore how we can create inclusive communities of people in different life stages, focusing on the concern of compromised cognitive conditions and on the potential of younger people to be mobilized to promote such a goal. While aging is frequently discussed from medical, economic, or technological perspectives, the Sharing Conversations project and its intergenerational haiku activity seek to highlight the significance of human interaction enhanced by a humanities-based activity.

Intergenerational Haiku-Making Activity: Activity Summary

The intergenerational haiku-making activity provides a platform for older people living with cognitive impairments and younger people to connect through collaborative poetry composition and communicate on an equal playing field. As noted in the Background section, a key strength of this activity lies in the imagistic nature of haiku, which can be composed using short phrases that describe emotional responses to natural scenes, making it free from the logical and grammatical constraints of prose. This structure enables a failure-free environment that engages participants' self-expression and imagination. Furthermore, while haiku follows a simple format and thus can be easily enjoyed by all age groups, it is also usually an unfamiliar form for English speakers, which reduces the advantage younger participants often have in other communicative settings and allows for more balanced and equal intergenerational interaction. This is further supplemented by the use of seasonal and personally meaningful pictures as a basis for composition, which reduces the need for memory retrieval by providing older participants a tangible object from which they can draw creative inspiration while still expressing aspects of their own identities.

Below we present the basic materials and steps needed to facilitate the intergenerational haiku-making activity for a group of six participants (i.e., three older and three younger). These may be tailored to fit an online format, as well as for groups of different sizes including one-on-one sessions between an older person living with dementia and their caregiver, in which case the latter would play the role of both facilitator and younger participant.

Materials

1. PowerPoint® slides for a ~10 min presentation that introduces the genre of haiku and prepares participants for the subsequent haiku-making and pair-work.
2. Three seasonal pictures in digital format in the slides or printed on paper, which participants can use as a basis for making their haiku.
3. A few haiku-writing sheets for participants to write their haiku on (e.g., 1-page Word document with 3 lines for the 5–7–5 haiku and a blank space for brainstorming).
4. Pencils or pens.
5. A means of showing the presentation slides (e.g., laptop, iPad, hard copies, TV, screen). This depends on where and with whom this activity is implemented.
6. A room with tables and chairs.

Optional: If the activity is done over Zoom® or other video conferencing platforms, devices (e.g., laptop, iPad) and headphones are needed.

Steps to Activity

1. Prior to the session, instruct participants to bring seasonal photos, ideally ones that are personally meaningful in some way. Alternatively, they may also choose from photos provided by the facilitators during the session.

2. Prepare a space for participants to gather, whether an open area in the healthcare facility such as the cafeteria or activities room or a more private space such as the residents' own rooms, depending on the desired scale. If done over Zoom®, each participant can join from their own room. Lay out writing paper, writing utensils, and the provided pictures at each table where participants will be seated.

3. The older participants (e.g., residents of the healthcare facility) and younger participants gather in the shared space and sit in pairs of older and younger.

4. The facilitators begin the activity session by introducing themselves with their name and their favorite season and reason why. Participants then introduce themselves with the same information. This self-introduction time (~5–10 min) can be used as an icebreaker by pointing out patterns in participants' favorite seasons, asking follow-up questions, or making comments on participants' answers, etc.

5. Facilitators begin the activity by introducing the genre of haiku through a brief (~10–12 min) interactive PowerPoint® presentation. In this section, emphasize the variety of possible interpretations of any topic/picture in order to minimize the pressure of making a "correct" haiku and highlight the participants' expressive freedom.

6. The presentation begins with a series of slides on "what is haiku," including a description of the genre and around three examples. For each example, include a relevant picture and an interactive question to mimic the activity's haiku-making format and engage participants. Facilitators can be creative with this section, for instance by choosing poems and pictures that fit the particular season/setting of the session, having participants make predictions about the picture from the poem or vice versa, etc.

7. Following this introduction, use one last example as a warm-up by having participants finish an incompletely shown haiku based on the picture paired with it. After hearing participants' ideas, reveal the original last line and compare it with everyone's lines to demonstrate how many different ways one can write a haiku on the same picture.

8. End the presentation with tips and guidelines for the participants' own brainstorming and writing.

9. Following the presentation, participants are given ~5 minutes to begin writing their own haiku, either based on the picture they have brought or on one of the provided pictures, which they can choose from at this time. Leave the tips and guidelines slide open on the screen/display for reference. Participants often finish at least one poem during this time and facilitators can encourage them to write more, but also stress that there is no pressure to finish even one poem, as they may continue it in the following segment with their partners.

10. Next, the facilitator announces the transition into the pair work segment (~15–20 min). In this segment, the first step is for each participant to finish one haiku if they have not already; let them know that they may help each other to do this. Once both poems are finished, participants share their poems and pictures with each other, including the stories behind the pictures and the thinking behind their poems. This often leads to deeper conversations beyond the haiku itself, though it differs with each pair. There are also many mini-activities that pairs can do if time is left, such as creating haiku on each other's images or working together to compose a poem. Have a PowerPoint® slide open with a list of possible conversation topics and mini-activities so that participants have a structure to fall back on in case they are not sure how to interact.

11. After the pair work segment, have everyone transition back into the full group to share their haiku poems and pictures, including both their own and any other poems created in their pairs (~10–15 min). Make sure that participants know they can share just as much as they are comfortable, and encourage everyone to ask questions or make comments on each other's poems, which facilitators can do first to set an example.

12. End the session with a thank you haiku from the facilitators. This is optional, but very fun and well-appreciated!

13. Take pictures of everyone's handwritten haiku and pictures before they leave so that facilitators can record the poems and turn them into a *haiga* (Japanese art form consisting of a picture paired with a haiku poem) collection. This can be shared as a pdf and/or as paper copies with the participants and their families, friends and caretakers, who can then display them within their residences or facilities as desired.

Reflection

Having facilitated and observed the haiku-making activity sessions, we have witnessed firsthand the process by which meaningful intergenerational connections are created between older participants living with cognitive impairments and younger participants. In their first encounter, they often only exchange greetings and a few words. However, as they work together in pairs and groups via the picture-based haiku-making, we see them laughing together and bonding over many things such as their favorite seasons, flowers, colors, activities, and even things that they are not fond of, like the texture of sand or bugs. In the younger-older pair interaction, the participants often talk about previous experiences and memories evoked by the seasonal pictures in addition to helping each other with their haiku. As they begin to talk and connect more deeply, they also physically lean towards each other and show their increasing engagement through their body language.

After each activity session, we ask participants about their experience. Their reflections reveal the positive impacts of the haiku-based younger–older pair interactions. Many of them expressed how enjoyable and evocative it was to be able to hear other people's perspectives through their poems and conversations. Participants also spoke about how haiku served as a "springboard to the conversation(s)," and how the resulting interactions broadened their perspectives and facilitated mutual understanding across generations and different backgrounds. Notably, these kinds of reflections and the wordings used were the same across the older and younger generations, showing how both groups benefited equally from the chance to interact with people outside of their own age group. For example, one older participant shared:

> I thought *the idea of a partnership* was—really, it *helped me a lot.* I think that was one of the key things. So much *more productive and evocative* than just one person? It was great. You just get ideas that you didn't think of, you know? The *other person's awareness or a way of seeing it was wonderful.* It was completely different [. . .] An old guy and a young girl, that was all good things. *More differences you get there, the better it is.* And they may find things in common despite the differences or things very different.

Younger participants also mentioned:

> I think, coming from, I guess, obviously, *rather different backgrounds, the ways that we look at things turned out to be really different,* even though we were looking at the same thing. And I think

that *being able to sort of articulate these differences* and pointing them out was . . . was really *interesting* for me.

I think having *a mix of ages and experiences* makes the conversations a lot more *interesting* [. . .] *From the haiku, you can learn a lot more about another person.*

We also witnessed how haiku-making using seasonal pictures increased sensory stimulation for older participants and enabled them to engage in self-expression, self-discovery and imagination. Many of them cited specific aspects of their pictures that they liked or noticed, such as roses, butterflies, or certain colors, while they engaged in the picture-based haiku-making. This then often led them to think of other memories and aspects of their lives, which they put into their poems. For instance, one older participant said:

[Looking at his picture] This looks *dry,* and that looks *wet.* Yeah, So I had to *bring that feeling into it.* Morning yellow, no moisture to spare. Obviously, they had to have some life to be had. They're going to get life no matter what. Determination, strength. And then ignoring the green leaves. What green leaves? And oh, hey, there are green leaves there. It's actually grass, but that's beside the point. *We're taking artistic license, right?*

Post-session reflections on this creative process were overwhelmingly positive as well, as shown subsequently. A number of participants even said that they plan to continue creating haiku going forward, showing how even a one-time activity session can have long-lasting positive effects.

It [picture-based haiku-making] *got me remembering things and experiences.* And the fact that I had seen this color green [in the picture]. And at a time when I was a student and I was studying a year in Denmark. And it just—phew, my life just blew up, and was related to that color green. It was so, ah, intense [. . .] I think *haiku was just kind of magical.* Once people realize that, which I realized, then you really want to go with it!

When participants share their poems, pictures, and the special stories behind them to the whole group after the pair interaction, they often exchange positive comments and compliments about each other's contributions. Each sharing always concludes with a warm round of applause and heartfelt appreciation from everyone attending the activity. These wholesome moments put a smile on the faces of the facilitators and observers, as well as the participants. Saying goodbye after each activity session inevitably gets harder for both younger and older participants.

Some say the session is too short, while others ask when they can see each other again. At in-person sessions, they usually continue interacting with each other as they prepare to leave the room.

We have received positive feedback from both participants and staff members of the assisted living and adult day services. Overall, people appreciate how this activity creates an opportunity to form meaningful intergenerational connections. This opportunity sometimes even leads younger participants to seek further volunteering opportunities with older adults in the community. Additionally, we have been told by staff members how this activity can increase sensory stimulation for older adults with cognitive impairments and promote their emotional well-being. In particular, this haiku-making activity can help them build their confidence in their abilities. Several older participants mentioned how they were initially hesitant to join the activity, as they expected it to be too hard for them, but once they actually started making haiku, they found it surprisingly fun, relaxing and easier than they had thought.

> [I thought] a haiku *would be very difficult,* very stressful to do. I wasn't looking forward to it, but it was—*it's kind of fun and it was easy,* and I guess, I did better than I thought I was gonna do. Probably the biggest thing is I was surprised, *I surprised myself.*

> I enjoy the atmosphere that you've succeeded in creating here. I don't know how you did it. *I didn't think it was going to be possible* when I first came in. But it was *like magic.* [. . .] When we started—when I first came in, I thought, *Oh no, I can't do this* but you just created, um you know, *feeling of being relaxed.* It was *like a miracle.*

In addition to the positive comments, we also received suggestions for improvements. Some older and younger participants who attended one-off sessions recommended a longer session as it would create more opportunities to interact with one another. For instance, an older participant mentioned, "I just—it would be nice to have [the session] a little longer," while a younger participant also shared, "I wish we had more time [. . .] And I wish we could have talked to the other group that was participating as well. Like, you know, just have more, like, cross pair interaction?" Given the feedback, the project team members concurred and subsequently designed and implemented a three-day session, as described in the Background section. We have been receiving positive feedback for the extended session. For instance, a younger participant who participated in both types of sessions told us that the one-off session felt quite short, and that he preferred the longer session. Similarly, some younger participants mentioned that they appreciated meeting the same people over three consecutive weeks, as it helped them form a stronger bond with their older partners.

Another point to note is the growth of student activity facilitators as more effective communicators with older adults living with cognitive impairments. Each facilitator learns how they can best communicate with the participants as they run the activity. One facilitator came to realize the importance of silence and patience, while another learned how to affirm, encourage, and ask questions to the participants in a way that fully accommodates their needs.

This has been a learning opportunity for us as well. The haiku and all the contributions from the older participants during the activity enabled us to move beyond our own ageism and ableism and led us to re-appreciate older adults living with cognitive impairments in their fullness—who they are as individuals and how they communicate with the world. The older participants' rich life experiences and perspectives are eloquently reflected in their haiku, and the quality of these poems surprises and impresses us every time. Sometimes, we hear about previous participants passing away afterwards, which further motivates us to create a meaningful space for their voices to be heard and preserved until their last moments of life. The formation of meaningful intergenerational connections between the participants offers us hope for a society that transcends the pervasive generational barriers and connects everyone regardless of their ages and cognitive conditions.

Conclusion

The participants' interactions during the activity and post-session reflections reveal that, as partly described in the Reflection section above and as shown in our study based on the online sessions (Matsumoto et al., 2023/2024), the format of small group haiku creation and appreciation facilitated self-expression and the sharing of personal narratives for both the older and younger participants. The activity impacted them positively by encouraging respectful and supportive interactions as equals across generations and cognitive conditions.

Giles et al. (1992) find that "young people generally have negative assumptions about communicating with older persons" (p. 292) and hypothesize that "older people engage in self-stereotyping processes" (p. 293). This feature associated with older people, however, was not observed in our activity. In contrast, Williams and Nussbaum (2001) state that intergenerational friendship can be established outside of family. Our study suggests that friendly and inclusive intergenerational interactions can be promoted when the setting of an activity expects equal participation and positioning. Social connection of persons in different life stages and with varied cognitive conditions may be fostered using structured designs and guidance in humanities-based activities.

Questions to Consider

1. If you were to facilitate the activity, what kinds of questions or prompts would you give to the participants to facilitate their self-expression and to spark meaningful conversations?
2. How would you create an inclusive environment for the activity?
3. How can you learn to ask leading questions?
4. How would you respond to sad/unpleasant feelings and memories shared by the participants?
5. How would you react when participants are having difficulty remembering things?
6. If you were to alter the activity, what would you change and why?
7. What are your 5 Big Takeaways from this chapter?

Resources

1. Stanford Sharing Conversations (https://sharingconversations.sites.stanford.edu/)
2. Alzheimer's Association (www.alz.org/)
3. Haiku Society of America (www.hsa-haiku.org/)
4. The Haiku Foundation (https://thehaikufoundation.org/)
5. P. Kocher (2008). "Their Capacity to Delight": Knowing persons with dementia through Haiku. Master's Thesis, Queen's University Canada. Available from the Haiku Foundation Digital Library (www.thehaikufoundation.org/omeka/items/show/1381)

Notes

1 The application was made in association with Melanie Vetter, Distinguished Career Institute at Stanford.
2 Harumi Maeda is currently a PhD student in Japanese linguistics and Emily Wan was an undergraduate majoring in Japanese literature at Stanford University. Wan is now a PhD student at Harvard University.

References

Beam, C. R., & Kim, A. J. (2020). Psychological sequelae of social isolation and loneliness might be a larger problem in young adults than older adults. *Psychological Trauma: Theory, Research, Practice, and Policy, 12*(S1), S58–S60. http://dx.doi.org/10.1037/tra0000774

Christiansen, J., Qualter, P., Friis, K., Pedersen, S.S., Lund, R., Andersen, C.M., Bekker-Jeppesen, M., & Lasgaard, M. (2021). Associations of loneliness and social isolation with physical and mental health among adolescents and young adults. *Perspectives in Public Health, 141*(4), 226–236. https://doi.org/10.1017/S0144686X19001338

Davis, B. H. (Ed.). (2005). *Alzheimer talk, text and context: Enhancing communication.* Palgrave Macmillan.

Giles, H., Coupland, N., Coupland, J., Williams, A., & Nussbaum, J. F. (1992). Intergenerational talk and communication with older people. *International Journal of Aging and Human Development, 34*(4), 271–297. https://doi.org/10.2190/TCMU-0U65-XTEH-B950

Guendouzi, J. A., & Müller, N. (2006). *Approaches to discourse in dementia.* Lawrence Erlbaum Associates.

Hamilton, H. E. (1994). *Conversations with an Alzheimer's patient: An interactional sociolinguistic study.* Cambridge University Press.

Hamilton, H. E. (2011). At the intersection of art, Alzheimer's disease, and discourse: Talk in the surround of paintings. In P. Backhaus (Ed.), *Communication in elderly care: Cross-cultural perspectives* (pp. 166–192). Continuum.

Hamilton, H. E. (2019). *Language, dementia and meaning making: Navigating challenges of cognition and face in everyday life.* Palgrave Macmillan.

Kitwood, T. (1997). *Dementia reconsidered: The person comes first.* Open University Press.

Matsumoto, Y. (2011). Painful to playful: Quotidian frames in the conversational discourse of older Japanese speakers. *Language in Society, 40*(5), 591–616. https://doi.org/10.1017/S0047404511000698

Matsumoto, Y. (2019). Taking the stance of quotidian in talking about pains: Resilience and defiance. *Linguistics Vanguard, 5*(s2). https://doi.org/10.1515/lingvan-2018-0034

Matsumoto, Y., Maeda, H., Wan, E., & Liao, H. (2023/2024). On an even playing field of haiku making: An inclusive activity of creative verbal art. *Pragmatics and Society, 15*(1), 104–121. https://doi.org/10.1075/ps.23037.mat

Pinkert, C., Kerstin Köhler, K., von Kutzleben, M., Hochgräber, I., Cavazzini, C., Völz, S., Palm, R., & Holle, B. (2021). Social inclusion of people with dementia: An integrative review of theoretical frameworks, methods and findings in empirical studies. *Ageing and Society, 41*(4), 773–793. https://doi.org/10.1017/S0144686X19001338

Ramanathan, V. (1997). *Alzheimer discourse: Some sociolinguistic dimensions.* Lawrence Erlbaum Associates.

Ryan, E. B., Byrne, K., Spykerman, H., & Orange, J. B. (2005). Evidencing Kitwood's personhood strategies: Conversation as care in dementia. In B. H. Davis (Ed.), *Alzheimer talk, text and context: Enhancing communication* (pp. 190–198). Palgrave Macmillan.

Williams, A., & Nussbaum, J. F. (2001). *Intergenerational communication across the life span.* Lawrence Erlbaum Associates.

6 Artist in Residence

An Intergenerational Living and Learning Program

Lorna E. Segall, Caroline Mwenda, Kaitlyn Beard and Mackenzie Leighty

---

Objectives

By the end of this chapter:

1. You will understand the benefits of intergenerational engagement of a living and learning program housed within a personal care facility.
2. You will learn about the Artist in Residence program as a model for college students and persons living with dementia, facility administrators and community members.
3. You will be able to identify ways of implementing modified versions of this program that fit within your resources and community.
4. You will understand the practical and logistical manner of implementing an AIR program.

Introduction

As advancements in medicine and technology expand the human lifespan, humans are finding themselves living longer, living better and, for some, this may require remaining in the workforce longer whether it be for financial, social and personal preference (AARP International, 2023). As a result, the work force is looking increasingly multigenerational, family composition is taking on an intergenerational tone, and opportunities for intergenerational engagement are increasing. Reframing what it means to age is crucial to promoting a positive narrative for all ages as ageist perspectives (discriminating based on one's age) can have harmful effects for us all. As of the writing of this chapter in the

DOI: 10.4324/9781003359463-8

spring of 2024, ageism is playing a role in the upcoming presidential election, with many voters debating whether age affects a candidate's ability to serve effectively. Perspectives on aging and the impacts of ageism have far-reaching consequences for individuals, culture and society. While ageism is often associated with older adults, it also affects young people (World Health Organization, n.d.).

"One of the biggest threats to reframing attitudes toward aging lies in the increasing age segregation of American society. We're in the midst of a dangerous experiment where young people have almost no contact with older people outside of intermittent contacts in their own families" (Pillemer, quoted in Weir, 2023). Finding ways for generations to engage plays a valuable role in understanding each other, building positive relationships and creating positive outcomes for society (Feyh, Clutter & Krok-Schoen, 2022). Intergenerational programming has shown promising results in countering the harmful effects of age discrimination and promoting the wellbeing of older adults (Zhong, Lee, Foster & Bian, 2022).

Broadly defined, intergenerational programming includes activities or exchange between any two generations that fosters feelings of cooperation and meaningful interaction (Giraudeau & Bailly, 2019). Examples of such engagement could include learning together, making music together, creating art, taking field trips, baking, or attending community concerts. Regardless of the activity, intergenerational programming enhances cognitive, social and health outcomes and combats ageism, yielding critical benefits for all participants (Krzeczkowska et al., 2021; Feyh et al., 2022; Lytle, Nowacek & Levy, 2020). Successful intergenerational engagements are relatable and feasible, seamlessly allowing different age groups to interact. The arts and humanities provide exciting opportunities for enhancing human engagement.

This chapter highlights an Artist in Residence: Intergenerational Living and Learning Program (AIR). The mission of the AIR program is to enrich the lives of young and older adults through music, intergenerational engagement and lifelong learning, in an effort to foster a sense of belonging and celebrate diversity for everyone. As noted in previous chapters of this text, isolation is the enemy to sustaining well-being, especially for those with limited autonomy, such as older adults, the incarcerated and caregivers. Maintaining meaningful relationships, staying physically active and remaining cognitively engaged are vital, yet challenging, for those who need it the most. Programs like AIR address these needs innovatively and can have lifelong, life changing impacts.

Background

Inspired by the 2006 documentary film *Andrew Jenks, Room 335* (see www.andrewjenks.com), the Artist in Residence program was created in 2019 by Dr. Lorna Segall, director of music therapy at the University of Louisville, in partnership with the personal care facility Presbyterian Homes and Services of Kentucky (PHSK). Each academic year, two music students from the University of Louisville's music therapy program move into PHSK full time, for free, in exchange for intergenerational programming. The AIRs share a room on the second floor of the facility and live within their grand neighbor community. Examples of engagement could include singing, technology support, gardening, field trips, baking, hanging around, sharing meals and songwriting. Students are encouraged to utilize their strengths and talents in designing activities, and to live their lives as normally as possible; whether that means holding study groups for upcoming exams, inviting friends over to hang out, or being picked up for a Friday night date.

For the facility residents, this program addresses their need for increased meaningful engagement, cognitive stimulation, mobility and the development of meaningful relationships. For the students, this experience enhances their future skill set as clinicians, demystifies aging, and also engages them in developing meaningful relationships. Both parties learn from one another and gain a deeper appreciation for those on the other end of the aging spectrum.

Facility administrators, healthcare workers and facility caregivers also experience meaningful relationships with the energetic AIRs. In some cases, the children of residents get to know the AIRs and become extended family members.

Benefits of an Artist in Residence Program

For the students:

- Demystify the older population/combat ageism
- Disseminate knowledge to others through lived experience
- Prepare for future clinical work through immersive learning
- Increase knowledge of self
- Experience being part of an expanded community of care/ grand neighbors
- Support housing needs

For the residents:

- Develop new relationships
- Make meaningful contributions/give back to the community
- Engage in creative activities

- Increase movement
- Promote cognitive engagement
- Combat ageism

For the healthcare staff:

- Enhanced work culture and satisfaction
- Meaningful relationships with the AIRs
- Indirect assistance with wellbeing of patients
- Unique work setting

For the administrators:

- Selling point for future residents/marketing tool
- AIRs provide additional support in the evening hours when fewer activity staff are working, thereby providing additional engagement and boosts community morale
- AIRS can be sounding boards for residents and provide active listening and support
- Comfort of having additional able-bodied, helpful individuals to provide perspective and support, and to enhance the care team
- Elevate morale for residents and staff

For the families:

- Knowing family members are receiving specialized care and additional attention

Perhaps one the most meaningful ways to communicate the impact of what an AIR program means for the students is shared below. The 2024/25 school year will be the fourth year of the AIR. Previous AIRS share their experiences below.

Caroline Mwenda

My senior year of college was shaping up to be the best yet, living with my best friend and meeting our new neighbors seemed exciting. I had no clue what I was getting myself into. Living in an assisted living facility as an AIR was not in my 5-year life plan. I was a poor college student, and the offer of free rent was hard to refuse. Little did I know, this program

*would be a transformative experience that shaped my character and my
career as a music therapist.*

As a music therapy student in university, I desired to work in geriatric populations. I thought if anything, this experience would make me
a better candidate for my future career plans. I did not expect to make
such meaningful and lasting friendships that continue to this day.

In an average week, we went to classes just like everyone else, came
home to play concerts on Sundays, invited in other musicians to perform at dinner time, played movies at night when all the staff had gone
home, and created different activities for the residents. My favorite moments though were sitting at dinner swapping stories and talking with
my friends or sitting in their rooms doing the same.

I came to realize that college students and geriatric populations often
exist in age-segregated bubbles apart from the rest of society. As an AIR,
we bridged gaps and made friendships, debated things we cared about,
offered wisdom and insight into each other's situations, grieved deaths
and decline of people we loved, attended funerals, celebrated birthdays
and bridal showers. And the most impactful part was that we were doing all of this together. The beauty of this program lies in its mundanity.
Playing board games, discussing the day's news, sharing meals—these
seemingly ordinary moments built genuine connections. This "intergenerational living" allowed us to truly integrate into each other's lives.

As a college student in a fast-paced music program, I was used to the
grind. My friends at PHSK taught me about what really matters in life.
Every single one of them said if they could go back in time, they would
spend more time with family and less time trying to get ahead. I learned
that if I was a little bit late to class because I was helping my friend move
a box she couldn't lift, my teachers would be okay. The slower pace of
life made space for genuine friendship. The residents threw me a bridal
shower and a going away party, brought me snacks and treats, and supported me in everything I did.

I did not realize how deeply painful it would be to leave my home
of 18 months, finish my internship and start a "normal life." I was so
used to having twenty-five grandparents (who knew more about me at
the time than my own grandparents did) asking questions like why I got
home so late, what did I have for dinner, if I could come play dominos
down the hall or whether I could help reconnect their Wi-Fi.

Now working professionally as a music therapist in the geriatric population, my experience at PHSK has been invaluable. As a young professional, companies want to know about your prior experience. My prior
experience wasn't just working but living among geriatric populations
which set me apart. This program fostered my empathy, bedside manner,
conversational skills, and ability to cultivate meaningful relationships. I am
grateful for this program and the innumerable ways it has shaped my life.

Mackenzie Leighty

Preparing for the program, I assumed it would be awkward and that my relationships with the residents would be superficial. Oh, how wrong I was. The friendships I formed were some of the deepest I had ever experienced, and they quickly became family. There was a deep connection, solid trust, and natural authenticity. I would love to say there were moments that I remember leading to the depth of these friendships, but in actuality it was an endless number of small, daily interactions that come from living life in close proximity with one another. There were, however, some specific moments that made the closeness most evident to me.

The first of these moments came on an evening where my roommate and I had a specific homework assignment that kept us in our room during dinner. About 30 minutes after we knew dinner had ended, we heard a knock at the door. One of our closest friends had come to check on us, asking about our absence and offering a strange Ziploc bag containing an unknown item. She explained that the portions at dinner were much too large (a common frustration from the residents) and they were worried about us missing dinner. So, she had packed up half of her baked potato and brought it to us, still warm. We thankfully accepted and giggled to ourselves about the way they consider us in everything. Not 10 minutes later, another knock at the door and another friend on the other side who go straight to business. She quickly handed us another Ziploc bag (now we understood what she was offering) and said she wanted to make sure we had eaten a warm dinner that night. Again, we offered our thanks and when the door shut, we burst out in laughter. These ladies sat at separate tables and without corresponding with each other, came to the same conclusion that they needed to put half their baked potatoes in Ziploc bags to ensure we had a warm dinner. This evening stood out as a specific time when my roommate and I realized how deeply they cared for us and how thankful we were for them.

Another moment that made me realize how close we had grown was when I went on a date (my first date with my now husband.) I hadn't told them I had a date, but as I sat with them at dinner, they started to question why I was dressed up. As I explained my reason, their excitement grew quickly. I told them he was picking me up shortly after their dinner finished to take me out to eat. I left to get my purse near the end of dinner and saw my friends at the table quietly talking to each other. When I came back, all the ladies I sat with at dinner were sitting in the lobby with chairs facing the door. They told me they wanted to see him when he came to pick me up, so they knew what he looked like. I will never forget the audience that sent me off on my date. And when I came back, those ladies were among the first people who heard how the date went. Almost two years later, when he proposed to me, those same ladies were among the first people to hear the news and see the ring.

My last memory that highlights the depth of relationship we experienced, is when I moved out. We had a party to send me off where I sang my final songs for them. I chose songs that were the most meaningful to me from our time together, one of which was "The Twelfth of Never" by Johnny Mathis. They introduced me to this song during one of our sing-alongs and it was the sweetest love song I had ever heard. As I sang, I couldn't help but cry because the love he describes in the song was what I felt for them. Moving out felt so much like moving out of my parents' house when I started college. The love and support they gave me created a home and a family that I was heartbroken to leave. They were forever in my heart. It was true then and it is true now: until the twelfth of never, I'll still be loving you.

Kaitlyn Beard

The Artists in Residence (AIR) program at the University of Louisville (UofL) had a great impact on my personal growth, career aspirations, and perspectives on aging populations. My interest in this type of experience began when Dr. Segall showed the film Andrew Jenks, Room 335 in one of my undergraduate music therapy classes. In this film, a young adult moved into an assisted living facility and filmed his experience of learning and experiencing life with older adults living in an assisted living facility in southwest Florida. This documentary sparked my interest in older adults. As I continued through my undergraduate career, I felt a calling to work with older adults as a music therapist. I sought out each opportunity possible to engage in music therapy clinical experiences with older adults and took great responsibility for my clinical and personal role in these communities. When Dr. Segall began presenting the idea of creating an opportunity for UofL music therapy students to move into an assisted living facility, I did not hesitate to engage. Because I was already familiar with the life experiences, joy, and wisdom these individuals had to share, I knew this experience would be life-changing for me. I was very lucky that a fellow peer and friend was also interested in participating. In the moment that this dream became a reality, Paige and I looked at each other and gave each other a nod of approval which indicated that we would be discussing this further after class ended. Paige Nagle and I were the first AIRs to move into the Rose Anna Hughes Home in the Fall of 2020.

I learned through this experience that not only was I interested in learning about their lives, but they were interested in learning about mine. From personal relationships to work schedules, they wanted to know everything! I have such precious memories of going on walks with a group of female residents in the parking lot each morning, playing music for a peaceful and positive atmosphere in the outdoor gazebo after walking, engaging in casual conversation and opportunities for genuine connection in the lobby, and providing spiritual music in the dining room with Paige on Sunday mornings. Living in a community where most of the population was 65 years of age and older was interesting in that I experienced a different pace of life. I learned to take life slower and admire the smaller things in life because life is so trivial, and we must live each day to the fullest. I was able to directly apply everything I was learning from this living environment into my personal relationships with my grandparents. I became more comfortable in interpersonal communication and increasingly more intrigued by learning about my own grandparents' life.

The patience and kindness of the facility residents and staff was inspiring. This program required a great deal of patience and kindness to allow two young undergraduate music therapy students to move into their facility with minimal expectations. The residents of the assisted living and skilled nursing facilities welcomed us with open arms during the COVID-19 pandemic and allowed us to be a part of their daily routines when it was not required of them. The staff members of the facility became some of the closest people in my life.

Because of this opportunity, I developed an ability to quickly connect and develop rapport with my patients and their families in my professional role as a board-certified music therapist. I continued to seek out learning opportunities through getting a master's degree in music therapy at Florida State University where I developed a similar AIR program paired with an experimental research study to measure the impact of intergenerational relationships through music on the biopsychosocial status of older adults residing in an assisted living facility.

This program was pivotal in my personal and professional life, and I highly recommend this experience to any individual looking to find purpose and joy in their life.

Establishing Your Own Artist in Residence Program

The goal of this activity is to provide the steps for initiating an AIR program in your community.

Steps to Initiating an Intergenerational Artist in Residence Program

1. Identify an enthusiastic collaborator in your community. This is the most crucial step. Enthusiasm on behalf of both parties is imperative. Other items to consider are geography and the physical space the AIRs will be living in.
2. Do you have a pool of students who may be interested? It is worth stating that while this program incorporates music students, it could be any creative student excited about participating in this experience. Examples of other meaningful areas of major could be creative writing, graphic design, dance, theater and even technology. Qualities of a successful AIR: genuine desire to participate, adaptability and flexibility, creativity and, perhaps most importantly, the AIRs are compatible. It has been my experience that each year, two students have already decided between themselves they want to participate together. This is such an important component to success. The AIRs must have a wonderful relationship as they will be leaning on each throughout their residency.
3. Identify someone at the facility to serve as a co-director who can also be an on-site point person for the AIRs.
4. Collaborate with your facility in designing the program. What will the requirements be for the AIRs? What are the various responsibilities of everyone's role? Remember to incorporate the strengths of the AIRs. This means that no two AIR residencies will be the same. It is important that the AIRs have autonomy in creating/implementing their activities while also having some structure is valuable and helpful, but too much structure is detrimental and uninspiring. Always remember: This is where the students live, and they must be comfortable. They shouldn't feel like they're "on the job" in their own home.

If developing an AIR program is not feasible, the section below offers ideas for programming modification. Resources section of this chapter for a list of program variations that may align with your community resources.

Modified Artist in Resident Intergenerational Programming

The chapter highlights the experience of music therapy students. This is primarily in part as the program creator also directs a music therapy program at the university. It is important to remember that the students living in these communities do not have to be music students. They could be a student engaged with any major (i.e. graphic design, communications, health sciences). Some intergenerational programs also exist incorporating adolescent aging out of foster care programs.

- Hosting a college class at a facility.
- Students could give final project presentations throughout the semester at the facility as an offshoot of lifelong learning programming.
- Incorporate facility residents as part of class assignments throughout the semester.
- Host several residents on campus for a college event such as a music concert, lecture, play, or sporting event.

Program Director Reflection—Lessons Learned

I think a lot about the students while they're living in the facility. Are they comfortable? Do they have all the resources they need? Do they feel supported and empowered? Do they have enough structure to feel confident, yet enough space to be creative? Their quality of life is crucial, but I strive to respect their boundaries and avoid overstepping. Whether I succeed in this, only the AIRs can truly say.

I am deeply grateful to the AIRs who have allowed me to be part of their journey. It is an honor for me. I learn so much from hearing about their experiences and seeing how they integrate into the community. Their stories are heartwarming and affirming, making you proud to be human. I know the students walk away with a lifetime of memories, and I, too, gain immensely from this experience—confirming that everyone who engages in this journey benefits. Even after students have moved out, occasional visits or phone calls with their "grand neighbors" still happen. They return to show off engagement rings, surprise with a "hello," share wedding photos, or announce the news of an upcoming baby.

Despite my constant efforts to anticipate the students' needs, there are always unforeseen challenges. Especially in the first year of the program, we were all very much learning together. The students were immersed in the moment, while I tried to stay a step ahead, often feeling a bit removed from their immediate experience. The first year of the AIR program was particularly challenging, as COVID-19 became part of our lives seven months after the students moved in. Navigating the many layers of the pandemic presented tremendous learning opportunities for all of us. I will never forget stopping by the facility to watch remote bingo, with the AIRs running from room to room, racing upstairs and downstairs, to read out the numbers and identify the winners. Despite the restrictions the pandemic required, the unexpected moments of joy and seeing the unstoppable-ness of human nature were significant. Moments of joy were also balanced with valleys of sadness.

The AIR residency involves many grief experiences for both students and residents. The most obvious grief experience is the loss of a grand neighbor. While everyone has a different experience with grief and loss, I cautiously speculate, and hope, that these young students have limited experience with losing a loved one. Many still have active relationships with their grandparents. Supporting their emotional and mental well-being during these times is crucial and an opportunity for knowledge and growth. There is also the anticipatory grief everyone feels as the residency approaches its end. Preparing residents, students, administrators, healthcare staff, and myself for the conclusion of an AIR residency cannot be ignored and must be thoughtfully planned. Expensive or complicated plans are not required. Events like final sing-alongs or creating a goodbye gift—something the AIRs can take with them—are perfect. This transition is clearly a time for grief as goodbyes are said, rooms are packed up, and cars are loaded as students head to their next adventure. The facility feels different in their absence. And although the AIRs move on, the residents remain. In one way I feel that the older adults are more equipped to navigate these experiences of closure, but I'm not sure a lifetime of this practice makes it any less heartfelt.

In the third year of the AIR program, the entire facility moved to a brand-new building. While the move offered many positives (brand new space, updated materials, better floor plan for residents, this transition elevated stress levels for many residents, some of whom had lived in the original building for 12 years. The anxiety, and accompanying feelings of grief, of moving to a new space were significant. The AIR in residence at that time was a game-changer, providing continuity, encouragement and resilient energy throughout the transition. Her support made all the difference in the wellbeing and adjustment of the residents.

As I write this, the 2024/25 AIRs are moving into their space, decorating and planning interventions for the residents. The residents are getting to know them, remembering their names, and learning more about them. The students, too, are on the brink of being fully immersed in the cast of characters at PHSK and preparing to take on their new roles as artists in residence. Although I've gleaned many lessons over the past several years, one thing I know for sure is that each residency is unique. I cannot wait to support them, learn from them, and watch the residents welcome them into their community.

Conclusion

Collaborations of this kind are profoundly meaningful for all participants, with engagement opportunities limited only by the participants. Intergenerational programming, regardless of its structure, offers diverse ways to combat isolation and loneliness while enhancing the quality of life for facility residents. For caregivers, both institutional and personal, the support provided by such programs is invaluable, especially given the high risk of burnout often associated with their roles. For participating students, these experiences shape their life perspectives and leave a lasting impact. These programs contribute not only to their personal well-being but also to their professional insight and effectiveness.

Internet Resources for Intergenerational Engagement

1. EngAGEd: www.engagingolderadults.org/external-resources# caregivers
2. Generations United: www.gu.org/resources/connecting-generations-strengthening-communities-a-toolkit-for-intergenerational-program-planners/
3. TimeSlips Creative Storytelling: www.timeslips.org/trainings/individual-training/families/
4. World Health Organization: www.who.int/publications/i/item/9789240070264
5. World Health Organization: Age Friendly World: https://extranet.who.int/agefriendlyworld/

Questions to Consider

1. Do you have time to direct an AIR program?
2. Do you think you have enough interested students that a program could occur each year? This is important as the residents anticipate new students and programming should have continuity.
3. What do you think some challenges for your students might be? How can you mitigate those challenges?
4. How could you survey students to see who might be interested?
5. What do you think potential program administrators would like to know?
6. How can programs like these address ageism and change perspectives about aging and dementia?
7. How do you prepare students for this type of programming?

References

AARP International (2023). Longevity: What does increasing life expectancy mean for the future of work? www.aarpinternational.org/initiatives/future-of-work/megatrends/longevity

Feyh, L., Clutter, J. E., & Krok-Schoen, J. L. (2022). Get WISE (Wellness through Intergenerational Social Engagement): An intergenerational summer program for children and long-term care residents. *Journal of Intergenerational Relationships*, *20*(3), 293–311. https://doi.org/10.1080/15350770.2021.1879706

Giraudeau, C. & Bailly, N. (2019). Intergenerational programs: What can school-age children and older people expect from them? A systematic review. *European Journal of Ageing*, *16*(3) 363–376. https://doi.org/10.1007/s10433-018-00497-4

Krzeczkowska, A., Spalding, D. M., McGeown, W. J., Gow, A. J., Carlson, M. C., & Nicholls, L. A. B., (2021). A systematic review of the impacts of intergenerational engagement on older adults' cognitive, social, and health outcomes. *Ageing Research Reviews*, November (71). https://doi.org/10.1016/j.arr.2021.101400.

Lytle, A., Nowacek, N., & Levy, S. R. (2020). Instapals: Reducing ageism by facilitating intergenerational contact and providing aging education. *Gerontology & Geriatrics Education*, *41*(3), 308–319. https://doi.org/10.1080/02701960.2020.1737047

Weir, K. (2023, March 1). Ageism is one of the last socially acceptable prejudices. Psychologists are working to change that. *Monitor on Psychology*, *54*(2). www.apa.org/monitor/2023/03/cover-new-concept-of-aging

World Health Organization. (n.d.) Ageism. www.who.int/health-topics/ageism#tab=tab_1

Zhong, S., Lee, C., Foster, M. J., & Bian, J. (2022). Intergenerational communities: A systematic literature review of intergenerational interactions and older adults' health-related outcomes, *Social Science & Medicine*, *264*. https://doi.org/10.1016/j.socscimed.2020.113374

7 The Power of Music through Intergenerational Dementia Choirs

Debra Sheets

Objectives

By the end of this chapter:

1. You will understand the benefits of intergenerational engagement in music and, specifically, group singing for older adults with memory issues and their care partners.
2. You will learn about the choral group Voices in Motion™ (ViM) as a model for operating an inclusive and intergenerational community-based choir for persons living with dementia and their care partners.
3. You will be able to locate or initiate a supportive choral group designated for older adults living with dementia and their care partners.
4. You will understand the theoretical and empirical benefits of community-based dementia choirs to help garner institutional support and ensure sustainability.

Introduction

This chapter introduces readers to Voices in Motion™ (ViM), an intergenerational community-based choir for persons living with dementia, their care partners and community members. ViM is a professionally directed choir designed to address dementia stigma through an intergenerational and inclusive choir program that culminates in public concerts. Thus, the purpose of such dementia choirs is to shift the dementia narrative from one of decline and hopelessness towards one of inclusion, contribution and connection. Choir participation focuses on the strengths that remain rather than the losses that are associated with dementia. These choirs offer an intergenerational and caring community

DOI: 10.4324/9781003359463-9

of support that enhances quality of life and well-being for both persons living with dementia and their care partners. Like many of the activities presented in this text, ViM choirs reduce social isolation and the consequential risks common to both persons with dementia and their caregivers with outcomes that include improving cognitive function, and reducing loneliness, anxiety and depression. This chapter highlights the benefits of inclusive dementia choirs, advocates for the feasible and cost-effective programming of such choirs and describes how to create community-based dementia choirs.

Context

The ViM choir was developed by an interdisciplinary team of researchers (i.e., nursing, psychology, sociology, music) at the University of Victoria, British Columbia, Canada. Their rigorous study was the first to investigate the impact of choir participation on persons with dementia and their care partners. The intergenerational focus was unique and presented the opportunity for additional social connections while also addressing dementia stigma among youth. Dementia is a major public health concern globally as population aging continues to accelerate. In 2024, over 600,000 Canadians have been diagnosed with dementia and by 2030, that number is expected to be over a million (Alzheimer Society of Canada, 2022). ViM was created to offer a joy-filled, supportive and meaningful choir experience for persons living with dementia and their care partners (see Voices in Motion, 2023). Singers also benefit from belonging to a caring and supportive intergenerational community in which connections occur naturally through a shared interest in singing together. Additionally, this research suggests that community-based dementia choirs increase socialization, enhance cognitive function, restore a sense of purpose and meaning, and address stigma by challenging perceptions of dementia. This chapter summarizes the physical and mental health benefits experienced by persons engaged in group singing activities, in general, and in the ViM program, specifically, along with guidance on finding or creating a choral group aimed at connecting community members living with dementia, their care partners and others.

Health Benefits of Social Singing

Engaging in social or group singing has significant physiological and emotional benefits. Group singing diminishes levels of perceived stress, in part by facilitating the body's regulation of cortisol (a stress hormone) (Harvey, 2020). Similarly, levels of oxytocin, a neuronal signaling molecule linked to the promotion of bonding and trust between individuals increases, facilitating a sense of connection to others during participation in group music-making (e.g., singing, playing instruments, dancing) (Keeler, 2015). Singing, specifically, has been linked to reductions in chronic pain and depression (Irons et al., 2020). A meta-analysis investigating findings from Australia, Brazil, China (Hong Kong SAR), Germany, India, Italy, the Netherlands, Spain, Sweden, Thailand, Turkey, the UK and the US demonstrated that persons with chronic health problems involved in music interventions (e.g., listening, singing, creating music) report significant positive changes in their quality of life (QoL) (McCrary et al., 2022).

Singing is associated with positive physiological and emotional benefits that include increased oxygen intake, better cardiorespiratory capabilities, stronger respiratory muscularity, and increases in neurotransmitter production linked to positive emotions (for reviews of literature see Daykin et al., 2018; Kang, Scholp & Jiang, 2018,). Social singing contributes to social bonding with others and overall happiness, diminished stress, better immune function and better nightly sleep (Moss et al., 2018). Participation in choirs is associated with improved quality of life (QOL) and well-being as well as reduced social isolation and loneliness among all choir members.

Benefits of Choir Participation for Persons Living with Dementia

ViM research (McDowell et al., 2023) found that the rate of cognitive decline in choir participants with dementia was about one-half what would be expected based on comparison with national dementia data. In the Vim study cognitive function was measured using the Mini Mental State Examination (MMSE) to assess delayed memory, attention, language, visuospatial ability, and orientation in time and space. Participants were tested approximately every month during the choir season, with some individuals being assessed up to 10 occasions over a 1.5-year period. Results show that, over the course of the study, rates of decline on the MMSE were significantly less compared to a national sample. The average ViM choir participant with dementia declined about 1.3 units per year on the MMSE, compared to other non-intervention studies where rates of decline were 2–3 times faster. This study highlights the meaningful impact of group singing on reducing social isolation, depression, anxiety and dementia stigma and its mitigating effects on cognitive function. Because social singing relies heavily on procedural and emotional memory, individuals with dementia are situated to successfully engage (Tamburri et al., 2019). This allows persons living with dementia to still fluidly sing despite progressive impairment in cognition and memory (2019, p. 76) (as also discussed in Chapter 6).

Researchers suggest that ViM members with dementia had reduced cognitive decline due to group singing, increased social connections and public concert performances. The act of engaging in social singing was meaningful, contributed to new friendships and a caring community. These findings underscore the benefits of social singing to protect against accelerated cognitive decline for persons living with dementia.

Benefits of Choir Participation for Care Partners of Persons Living with Dementia

Care partners also benefit from participation in community-based dementia choirs with their family member living with dementia. Osman and colleagues (2016) studied patient–carer pairs residing in the East Midlands area of the United Kingdom, who participated in *Singing for the Brain*, a therapeutic music program that involves the care partner, the care recipient with memory loss, and a musician singing familiar songs that follow a different theme each week. Six themes were identified from the data that can inform the importance of dementia music programs (Osman et al., 2016, p. 1330):

1. Social inclusion and support.
2. A shared experience.
3. Positive impact on relationships.
4. Positive impact on memory.
5. Lifting the spirits.
6. Acceptance of the diagnosis.

Similarly, Smith and colleagues (2022) find parallel benefits to both care partners and the family member living with dementia who were members of ViM. Their study finds that both care partners and persons living with dementia, as well as the students, experienced transformative

Table 7.1 ViM health benefits

Health benefit	Measure	Source(s)
Helps slow or stabilize general cognition and perceptual speed	MMSE TMTA	Tamburri et al., 2019
Social benefit		
Mitigates anxiety and depression	PHQ-9	Tamburri et al., 2019
Decreases social isolation and loneliness	PHQ-9	Tamburri et al., 2019

Notes: MMSE = Mini-mental State Examination (Folstein, Folstein & McHugh, 1975); TMTA = Trail Making Task A (Lezak, 1995); PHQ-9 = Patient Health Questionnaire (Kroenke, Spitzer & Williams, 2002).

benefits through the joy they experienced performing, the meaningful relationships that resulted and the ways in which they challenged the social stigma of dementia (Smith et al., 2022, p. 4). The specific health benefits resulting from participation in ViM are summarized in Table 7.1.

Benefits for Students Engaged in Voices in Motion

Students involved in a community-based choir experience similar positive benefits in social connections and well-being (Harvey, 2020; Irons et al., 2020; Keeler, 2015). However, Smith and colleagues (2022) show that students engaged in ViM experienced additional benefits. Specifically, the ViM students gained a better understanding of dementia, empathy for those with dementia, and positive relational experiences and friendships that challenged dementia stigma. Qualitative interviews with participants (Smith et al., 2022) demonstrate the personal and interpersonal benefits for all groups (i.e., care partners, persons with dementia, students) participating in the ViM choir.

Persons Living with Dementia

People really make an effort to address you by name and get to know you and, you know, it's not just about the choir and the singing. It's about the personal side as well.

(Smith et al., 2022, p. 5)

It's probably the best thing that's happened to me since I've lost most of it up here, you know, gradually. And so anyway, I'm losing that but still I'm gaining, gaining the singing that I had to stop with the Choral Society. And also, I was with two other choirs as well. And I just couldn't continue with them.

(Smith et al., 2022, p. 4)

When you have that enthusiasm, you're not doom and gloom, you know, you're singing with your whole body, your everything, and that spirit is in there you know. It's there and it's lifting you up, you know. That's a wonderful thing for us to have that happen because it makes us realize how human we are.

(Smith et al., 2022, p. 4)

Care Partners of Persons Living with Dementia

I think a lot of the couples are looking for the same thing—an outlet that they can be themselves and be treated with dignity.

And be part of something that they're actually doing, something constructive.

(Smith et al., 2022, p. 5)

[T]he friendship that ensues, that's a part of our life now.

(Smith et al., 2022, p. 5)

Community Members

[I]t's much more than a choir . . . it's a family of people, like people of all ages, and you can just chat with whoever you want to.

(Smith et al., 2022, p. 5)

There wasn't really much connection in like the first couple of rehearsals but then gradually as we got more comfortable with each other and as the music things got better, the connections were made and they became pretty strong by the end.

(Smith et al., 2022, p. 5)

Many of the participants—care partners and students—also spoke about the ways in which the choir changed their perspectives:

In the beginning you're always just thinking in the bottom of your head they have Alzheimer's so you should be careful with what you say so they won't be so confused . . . but as weeks progressed you start to forget that they have Alzheimer's and like the beginning of rehearsals you're just like, "Oh hey come sit with me" and you start chatting with them and it's more comfortable being with them.

(Smith et al., 2022, p. 5)

I think that the fact that we're on stage performing and people come from all walks of life, probably, come to hear us sing. And I'm sure they're observing us, hearing us, observing us and it probably does shift a few attitudes. And I think that's good. I think that's great! It's, yeah, just to be out, out in the world.

(Smith et al., 2022, p. 6)

I feel like all of us, you know, even for me when we first started, everyone kind of goes in with the same vision of what Alzheimer's is. Like, what's the point? Like they're just going to forget. But for me now, like if I ever hear someone talking about someone with Alzheimer's like that, I'd be like, "No, that's false. That's not right. Like it's completely opposite of that."

(Smith et al., 2022, p. 6)

The reflection from students suggests that the choir is effective in countering dementia stigma. Additionally, the choir is effective at bringing people together to mitigate the overwhelming epidemic of loneliness and isolation and the negative health consequences resulting from them.

Audience Members

Present research also demonstrates the benefits experienced by audience members attending live music venues. In 2005, a commission of 14 major universities arts presenters (MUP) launched the study *Assessing the Intrinsic Impacts of a Live Performance* as part of a larger multi-method collaborative research effort called *The Values and Impact Study* (Brown & Novak-Leonard, 2008).[1] Among their findings was evidence on the impact of live performances for individual audience members, and these positive findings have implications for viewers of ViM (and like performances). First, audience members report being intellectually stimulated as the performance aroused questions about the performance itself and the meaningfulness of the works performed (i.e., 42% reported questions arising while watching the performance, Brown & Novak-Leonard, 2008, p. 12). For ViM performances, this effect could very well raise social awareness and work to counter preconceptions of dementia, persons with dementia and care partner roles. The study also showed that audience members experience strong emotional responses that continued to resonate long after the performance ended (i.e., 54% reported lingering emotional resonance, Brown & Novak-Leonard, 2008, p. 13). More importantly, audience members report feelings of empathy towards one or more of the performers (Brown & Novak-Leonard, 2008. p. 13) which speaks directly toward the social awareness goals of ViM, specifically, to change social biases toward and increase empathy for persons living with dementia. Lastly, the study reports live performances help cohere social bonds: "On an interpersonal level, arts experiences deliver social impacts as well, in the form of family cohesion, expanded social networks and an enhanced ability to empathize with others" (Brown & Novak-Leonard, 2008, p. 14). A 2023 study on audience effects of support concerts is also hopeful. Williams and colleagues report:

> Our results provide new evidence of the audience's responses to amateur choir performances, by demonstrating that witnessing both community and recovery choir performances can foster admiration, respect, and positive regard toward choristers regardless of their mental health status.
>
> (Williams et al., 2023, p. 1537)

These findings are encouraging that ViM, and other such, concerts are affecting changes to societal views on dementia with each participant and each audience member.

Convening a Voices in Motion™ Group: Activity 1 Summary

The goal of this activity is to provide the steps for initiating an intergenerational dementia choir in your area.

Steps to organizing a ViM Chior

1. Measure your community's need and participant interest: Survey local residential or senior centers, dementia support groups, geriatric clinics, or churches.
2. Do you have at least 10 duets (couples) able to participate and 5 students interested in being involved?
3. Identify a host organization: Are there any existing community-based intergenerational choirs? Alternatively, is there an organization that would welcome adding an intergenerational choir?
4. Locate personnel and resources: Who needs to be on your leadership team? What resources do you have to help fund a choir director and operational costs?
5. Clearly and comprehensively design your program: What are the objectives? How will you recruit? What area will be served? How will the program be funded? Where will the program be held (e.g. consider accessibility, size, lighting, restrooms)? Who will provide administrative support?

If developing a new *dementia choir* is not feasible, please see the Resources section of this chapter for a list of additional music programs to locate a program nearest to you.

Convening an Intergenerational and Inclusive Dementia Choir: Activity 2 Summary

If no established intergenerational and inclusive dementia choir exists in your area, the following guidance provides directions on starting a dementia choir to engage persons living with dementia, older persons, care partners and students in a professionally directed choir.

Additional Help

Contact local colleges and universities, particularly those with music therapy programs to inquire about initiating a music or group singing program with undergraduate and graduate students to serve as the conveners of a musical program for persons living with dementia, their care partners, college students and community members. See also Chapters 6 and 9 for guidance on involving college student organizations and groups.

Reflection

A number of lessons can be drawn in considering how to develop an intergenerational and inclusive dementia choir. First, the personality of the professional choir director is crucial to make the choir fun, challenging and achievable. The choir director must also be comfortable helping people to get to know one another through all choir activities. Second, choirs need administrative support to help with recruitment, concert planning, photocopying, collating music notebooks, coordinating volunteers, organizing refreshments and more. Third, a carefully selected board of directors is critical to the long-term sustainability of these choirs and to reflecting participant preferences in decision-making. Fourth, well-chosen partnerships (e.g., high schools, Alzheimer's associations, caregiver organizations, college organizations, churches) can enrich and support these choir programs. Fifth, a few passionate people can make dementia choirs happen in their own communities. These programs are socially compelling and their positive impact on health and well-being, as well as overall community vitality, is supported by a growing body of research, for all who participate. Moreover, a growing network of dementia choir programs are creating a thriving social movement as new programs grow. In broader psychosocial terms, we are seeing choir programs like these promoting the vital involvement that Erikson and colleagues have defined as meaningful, reciprocal engagement between self and outside environment (Erikson et al., 1994; Kivnick & Wells, 2014); these scholars have identified *vital involvement* as the fundamental dynamic for creating and maintaining psychosocial health while facing changing abilities in later life.

Conclusion

An inclusive community-based dementia choir offers all participants an opportunity to learn, participate and experience joy together in a supported activity. The network of support and engagement that a community setting provides helps ameliorate the physical and mental health consequences of isolation and loneliness (for an extensive review on the effects of group activities for persons living with dementia, see Vedel et al., 2020). Participants also retain or regain an identity demonstrating their abilities to learn, to express themselves, and to be part of a socially meaningful activity. The low cost of establishing a community-based choir makes these programs attractive non-pharmacological interventions, particularly given the lack of a cure for Alzheimer's disease and related disorders.

Questions to Consider

1. Which aspects of belonging to an inclusive community-based dementia choir do you expect to be most rewarding for care partners? Persons living with dementia? Students?
2. What steps can you take to ensure that each population gets the most out of their participation?
3. Which considerations are key to ensuring the success of a dementia choir and might pose the most challenges, either in planning or in execution? What steps can you take to pre-empt or mitigate those challenges?
4. How might you present any of the above activities to program administrators or funding sources to secure their support?
5. Why should the choir be professionally directed with three-part (or more) harmonies?
6. How can student participation in these choirs reduce dementia stigma and contribute to a change in society-wide attitudes about dementia and aging?
7. What kind of training do students need to be most prepared to meaningfully engage with this population?
8. Why is a public concert an important part of the program for the choir? To further extend the activities described in this chapter, what kinds of sources (films, books, songs, news sources, etc.) might pair well with Shakespeare excerpts in commonplace books?

Resources

1. Voices in Motion: https://voicesinmotionchoirs.org/
2. Singing for the Brain: https://forum.alzheimers.org.uk/threads/what-is-singing-for-the-brain.87418 (singing support groups for persons with dementia in the UK)

3. Forget Me Not: www.forgetmenotchorus.com (singing support groups for persons living with dementia in the UK)
4. Giving Voice: https://givingvoicechorus.org/for-singers/u-s-choruses (limited directory of US choirs for persons living with dementia)
5. Giving Voice limited directory of worldwide choirs for persons living with dementia: https://givingvoicechorus.org/for-singers/worldwide-choruses/

Note

1 Lead universities: University of Florida Performing Arts, Gainesville; University Musical Society, Ann Arbor, Michigan; Clarice Smith Performing Arts Center, University of Maryland; Lied Center for Performing Arts, University of Nebraska–Lincoln; Mondavi Center for the Performing Arts, University of California–Davis; ASU Gammage, Tempe, Arizona. Associate partners: Annenberg Center for the Performing Arts, University of Pennsylvania; Cal Performances, University of California–Berkeley; Center for the Performing Arts, The Pennsylvania State University; Hancher Auditorium, University of Iowa; Hopkins Center for the Arts, Dartmouth College; Krannert Center for the Performing Arts, University of Illinois; Lied Center of Kansas, University of Kansas–Lawrence; Stanford Lively Arts, Stanford University; Ontario Presenters Network.

References

Alzheimer Society of Canada. (2022). Navigating the Path Forward for Dementia in Canada: The Landmark Study Report# 1. https://alzheimer.ca/sites/default/files/documents/Landmark-Study-Report-1-Path_Alzheimer-Society-Canada.pdf.

Brown, A. S., & Novak-Leonard, J. L. (2008). Assessing the intrinsic impacts of a live performance. https://wolfbrown.com/insights/reports/assessing-the-intrinsic-impacts-of-a-live-performance/

Daykin, N., Mansfield, L., Meads, C., Julier, G., Tomlinson, A., Payne, A., Grigsby Duffy, L., Lane, J., D'Innocenzo, G., Burnett, A., & Kay, T. (2018). What works for wellbeing? A systematic review of wellbeing outcomes for music and singing in adults. Perspectives in Public Health. *138*(1), 39–46.

Erikson, E. H., Erikson, J. M., & Kivnick, H. Q. (1994). *Vital involvement in old age*. W. W. Norton & Company.

Folstein, M. F., Folstein, S. E., & McHugh, P. R. (1975). "Mini-mental state": A practical method for grading the cognitive state of patients for the clinician. Journal of Psychiatric Research, *12*(3), 189–198.

Harvey, A. R. (2020). Links between the neurobiology of oxytocin and human musicality. *Frontiers in Human Neuroscience, 14*, https://doi.org/10.3389/fnhum.2020.00350

Irons, J. Y., Sheffield, D., Ballington, F., & Stewart, D. E. (2020). A systematic review on the effects of group singing on persistent pain in people with long-term health conditions. *European Journal of Pain, 24*(1), 71–90.

Kang, J., Scholp, A., & Jiang, J. J. (2018). A review of the physiological effects and mechanisms of singing. *Journal of Voice, 32*(4), 390–395.

Keeler, J. R., Roth, E. A., Neuser, B. L., Spitsbergen, J. M., Waters, D. J. M., & Vianney, J. M. (2015). The neurochemistry and social flow of singing: Bonding and oxytocin. *Frontiers in Human Neuroscience, 9*, https://doi.org/10.3389/fnhum.2015.00518

Kivnick, H. Q., & Wells, C. K. (2014). Untapped richness in Erik H. Erikson's rootstock. *The Gerontologist, 54*(1), 40–50.

Kroenke, K., Spitzer, R. L., & Williams, J. B. (2002). The PHQ-15: validity of a new measure for evaluating the severity of somatic symptoms. *Psychosomatic Medicine, 64*(2), 258–266.

Lezak, M. D. (1995). Executive functions and motor performance. In M. D. Lezak (Ed.), *Neuropsychological Assessment* (3rd edition) (pp. 650–685). Oxford University Press.

McCrary, J. M., Altenmüller, E., Kretschmer, C., & Scholz, D. S. (2022). Association of music interventions with health-related quality of life: A systematic review and meta-analysis. *JAMA Network Open, 5*(3), e223236.

McDowell, C., Tamburri, N., Smith, A. P., Dujela, C., Sheets, D. J., & MacDonald, S. W. (2023). Exploring the impact of community-based choral participation on cognitive function and well-being for persons with dementia: evidence from the *Voices in Motion* project. *Aging & Mental Health, 27*(5), 930–937.

Moss, H., Lynch, J., & O'Donoghue, J. (2018). Exploring the perceived health benefits of singing in a choir: an international cross-sectional mixed-methods study. *Perspectives in Public Health, 138*(3), 160–168.

Osman, S. E., Tischler, V., & Schneider, J. (2016). "Singing for the brain": A qualitative study exploring the health and well-being benefits of singing for people with dementia and their carers. *Dementia, 15*(6), 1326–1339.

Smith, A. P., Kampen, R., Erb, T., MacDonald, S. W., & Sheets, D. J. (2022). Choral singing and dementia: Exploring musicality as embodied and relational accomplishment. *Journal of Aging Studies, 63*, 101077.

Tamburri, N., Trites, M., Sheets, D., Smith, A., & MacDonald, S. (2019). The Promise of intergenerational choir for improving psychosocial and cognitive health for those with dementia: The *Voices in Motion* project. *The Arbutus Review, 10*(1), 66–82.

Vedel, I., Sheets, D., McAiney, C., Clare, L., Brodaty, H., Mann, J., Anderson, N., Liu-Ambrose, T., Rojas-Rozo, L., Loftus, L., Gauthier, S., & Sivananthan, S. (2020). CCCDTD5: Individual and community-based psychosocial and other non-pharmacological interventions to support persons living with dementia and their caregivers. *Alzheimer's & Dementia: Translational Research & Clinical Interventions*, 6(1), e12086.

Voices in Motion. (2023). Join the movement. https://voicesinmotion-choirs.org/#:~:text=Voices%20in%20Motion%20is%20a,many%20 have%20been%20 life%2d Changing

Williams, E., Jetten, J., & Dingle, G. A. (2023). Audiences' emotional response to choir singing by people living with mental health conditions. *Psychology of Music*, 51(6), 1537–1552.

8 Bingocize®

Innervating Exercise through the Socialization Effects of Game

K. Jason Crandall

Objectives

By the end of this chapter:

1. You are expected to better understand the health benefits of tandem activities that combine physical exercise with cognitive tasks for older persons.
2. Specifically, you will learn about Bingocize®, a dual exercise program offered at many residential centers and through an online app.
3. You should be able to locate or request Bingocize® for the persons in your care.
4. You should be able to provide a rationale for requesting Bingocize® based on empirical support provided in this chapter.
5. You should be able to employ the principles of Bingocize® in activities that will achieve similar effects.

Introduction

Bingocize® is a socially engaging group-based program that combines exercise and health education with the widely popular game of bingo. It was created to address one of the most pressing health issues facing the elderly population: falls. Over 13 million adults 65 years of age and older will fall this year resulting in over $50 billion in health care costs (CDC, 2023). Borne out of the effort to decrease falls within the older population by increasing physical activity, (author) Crandall combined the common, long-term residential game of Bingo with whole-body engagement. The efficacy of this approach to curb falls, as discussed in the Context section below, generated an overwhelming adoption of Bingocize® in residential centers, which is now provided in centers within 47

DOI: 10.4324/9781003359463-10

US states, with additional sites also in Canada, Poland, and the UK In this chapter, I discuss additional health—physical and mental—benefits of Bingocize® as well as the general principles that have made Bingocize®'s combination of physical activity, cognitive tasks, and social engagement a boon for the health and wellbeing of its participants. The goal of this chapter is to further spread the availability of Bingocize® to the home-bound elderly, within residential centers, senior centers, trauma units, homebound, and, with hope, to the growing geriatric population within our prison systems. Additionally, if Bingocize® is unavailable or unat-tainable for some, this chapter provides guidance to readers to enact the general principles and, consequently, the health benefits of game-based activities that involve both physical and mental engagement for older persons and, particularly, those with neurological decline living in vari-ous environments.

The Connection of Bingocize® and Health Humanities

Some readers may be curious as to the inclusion of this chapter on an exercise program that is combined with the common game of Bingo in a collection grounded in health humanities. I present the case that rec-reational activities, including games and the practice of sport and ex-ercise, when used to promote physical, mental, and social health and wellness belong to the field of health humanities. I briefly present sum-maries of the theories, research, and academic efforts that support our view. The study of sport, game, and exercise has largely fallen under the theories of health, medicine, and sociology. Yet, at the turn of the twenty-first century the propensity of people to participate in sport, game, and exercise and the effects of such activities—their meaning and roles in the lives of human beings rather than at the larger societal level—was examined through a humanities lens (Basiaga-Pasternak & Blecharz, 2021; Kelly et al., 2019). This new lens allows such ac-tivities to be seen as part of the creative, philosophical, epistemologi-cal, and ethical aspects of human experience, all which contribute to the self-actualization of the individual. By extension, viewing sport, game, and exercise as part of the human experience—like we do art, literature, music—helps us answer questions of what it means to be human and what it means to live a meaningful existence. Such activi-ties contribute to our physical and mental health well-being and, as such, they may be examined within the theories of health humani-ties (see, for example, Soulé, Marchant & Verchère, 2022). Precisely since this text focuses on ensuring better situations for the elderly, humanities-driven questions such as how we may live meaningful lives—day by day—make this work an exceptionally fitted chapter to this collection.

Context

What is Bingocize®?

Bingocize® is an evidence-based health promotion program, designed by an exercise physiologist, that combines the familiar (and global) game Bingo with exercise and health education, specifically falls prevention, nutrition, and immune health information.

Bingo

According to the National Bingo Game (2024), the game Bingo originated in Italy around 1530 as a type of lottery that developed into a social, group game called *Beano*. Beano was brought to the US by toy salesman Edwin S. Lowe in 1929. Upon playing the game with friends, as the story goes, a participant yelled out "Bingo!" upon winning, and the modern version began its evolution. Presently, Bingo's rules of play are as follows (National Bingo Game, 2024):

1. Game participants are provided cards with five rows and five columns featuring 90, 85 or 75 numbers (the National Bingo Game is played using a set of 90 numbers, 1–90) with the word BINGO located at the top of each card (see Figure 8.1).

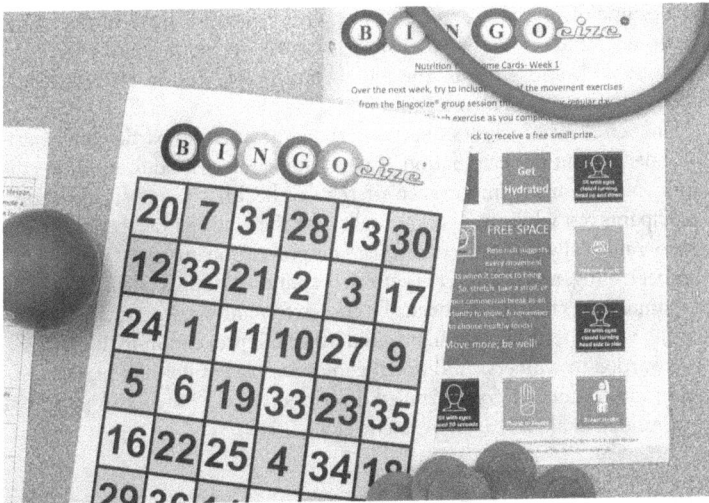

Figure 8.1 Bingocize® card

Source: Mark Schafer

2. A facilitator retracts a number from a container (usually a drum) that houses balls or chips with each number (e.g., 1–90) and announces the number.
3. If the number appears on a participant's card, then the participant marks the space of that number.
4. As participants mark numbers under each letter of the word BINGO, the first participant to spell out BINGO wins that round. Participants often win prizes, usually monetary rewards.

The National Bingo Game (2024) states that 8% of the UK population plays Bingo regularly, and Center Stage Artists (2024) claim that there are over 60 million Bingo players in the US. The ease of play, the entertainment and social benefits, and the opportunity to win prizes have made Bingo a popular game in communities (e.g., churches, drinking establishments, schools). These factors have also made the game a standard activity within long-term residential centers (Tak et al., 2015), and as such, the game provided the perfect activity to pair with physical exercise in the creation of Bingocize®.

Bingocize®

Bingocize® strategically combines the familiar game of bingo, falls prevention education, and exercise. Participants complete a series of strategically inserted exercises designed to increase or decrease the intensity and volume of exercise. Examples of exercises include head turns, trunk rotations, hand exercises focusing on grip strength, and extremity stretches with and without the aid of bands (see Figures 8.2 and 8.3, taken from an actual Bingocize® event).

Bingocize® also includes questions aimed at teaching participants valuable falls prevention information, such as home safety modifications, medication management, importance of regular health checkups, and more. Participants rest while numbers are called for the bingo game, then complete more strategically inserted exercises or falls prevention questions, rest during number calling, and so on. This pattern is continued until a participant wins the game. Prizes that are strategically chosen to reinforce the curriculum, including water bottles, night lights, and other fall prevention-focused items, are awarded to winners. Additional games are played until all planned exercises are completed (for a detailed description of the Bingocize® program, see Crandall et al., 2015; Dispennette et al., 2019).

Origin

Bingocize® began in the search for a physical based activity that would serve to increase balance and overall physical fitness to reduce falls in

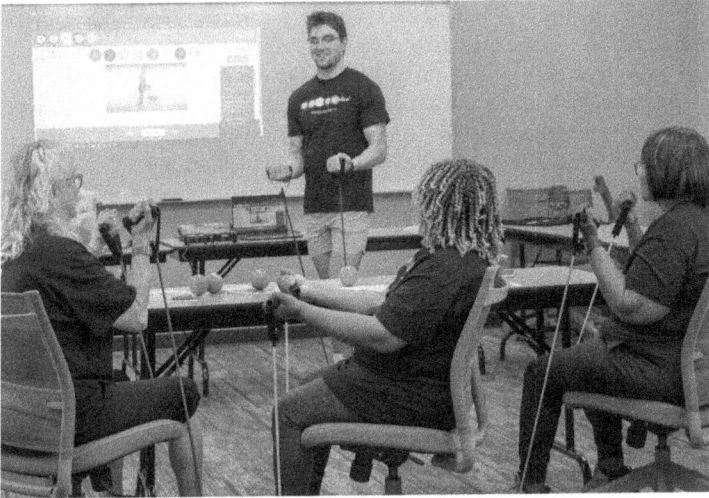

Figure 8.2 Extremity stretches from a Bingocize® event

Source: Mark Schafer

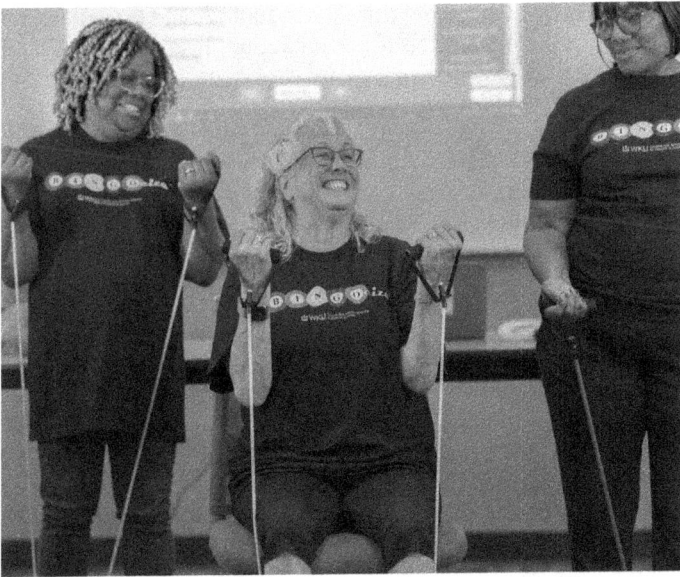

Figure 8.3 Extremity stretches from a Bingocize® event

Source: Mark Schafer

persons living within long-term residential centers. The concept origi-nated with the author, Dr. Jason Crandall; however, the idea for Bingo-cize® was truly a combination of serendipity and insight from one of my course assignments. A proponent of the pedagogy of service-learning, I asked my Exercise Science students to create an exercise program for older adults residing in an independent living facility close to the univer-sity and with whom the students were interacting as part of the course. Although the students followed instructions, no older adults attended the first session. After debriefing with the students, I discovered that the older adults were all playing Bingo in another part of the facility, preventing them from attending the exercise activities designed by the students. With the realization of the importance and popularity of Bingo within this and other residential facilities, I then decided to combine the game of Bingo with exercise.

Impetus: Health Consequences of Falls

A myriad of health consequences results from falls. Peels et al. (2019), in their meta-analysis on the health consequence of falls, notes that 33% require medical attention, with 5.7% result in fracture, 7.2% result in major injury, and 5% continue to suffer from their injury/ies one year later. Oliver and colleagues (2008) found that after a fall, even minor injuries can lead to rehabilitation, loss of confidence, in-creased fear of falling, and an increase in persons being moved perma-nently to residential centers.

As discussed above, most falls (i.e., 67%; Peels et al., 2019) do not result in immediate serious injury; however, it is worth noting the holistic impact or hip injury on daily activities. According to Komisar and colleagues (2022), the highest probability of injury from a fall occurs to the hip or pelvis region. Upon a review of the post-fall hip consequences, Marks and colleagues (2003) report that hip injury includes increased and expedited mortality, difficulty walking, and conducting daily activities, which then lead to, or exac-erbate, other issues such as cardiovascular health. Also, a hip injury will likely lead to a first-time admittance to a residential center, and many will begin the journey of long-term residence. Similarly, the next common fall injuries in the order of probability are those to the torso and shoulder, the elbow and forearm, the wrist and hand, knee, and, finally, head (for statistical data see Komisar et al., 2022). Each possibly leading to long-term or continual negative health and quality of life issues.

Impetus: Economic Costs of Falls

Corresponding to the health consequences of falls, the resulting medical costs are great and, as such, cannot be dismissed. According to the CDC, the economic cost resulting from falls for the year 2024 is expected to be $50 billion (CDC, 2024). Since falls in older adults account for both health and economic costs, the search for interventions to prevent their occurrence is one of the greatest concerns facing the geriatric medical community (Appeadu & Bordoni, 2023). To the goal of reducing falls in the elderly and the costs from falls, Bingocize® has inspired much hope.

Benefits of Bingocize®

Bingocize® is an Evidence-Based Fall Prevention Program (EBFP) approved by the National Council on Aging (NCOA) and the United States Department of Agriculture, and as such, a wealth of supportive study findings exists. Additionally, research findings continue to grow each year, strengthening the argument for including Bingocize® as part of the routine activities within community and residential centers across the globe. Additionally, the development of the Bingocize® web-based app, discussed later in this chapter, has made the Bingocize® available to the in-home elderly population as well as those in other living environments (see Figure 8.4).

Reduction in Fear of Falling

While many elderly embrace the idea of physical exercise and its health benefits, many refrain from engaging in such activity for fear that an injury may result; older persons report that their biggest fear is the health consequences and immobility they imagine from falling, making fear of falling the greatest predictor for inactivity for those aged

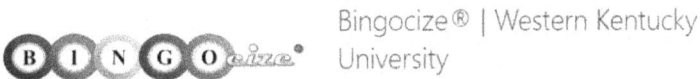

Figure 8.4 Bingocize® logo
Source: Mark Schafer

65 and older (Bertera & Bertera, 2008). Schafer et al. (2023, p. 1136) report that participants reported a significant reduction in their fear of falling after a 10-week adherence to Bingocize® (p = > 0.001; Cohen's d = 0.178). The greater implication of this finding is that a reduction in fear of falling can break the cycle between the fear of falling and the consequential reluctance to participate in physical activity. Once this connection is severed or at least significantly reduced, older persons are more likely to exercise or, simply, increase their daily activities, resulting in better overall balance and health, and leading to an actual reduction in falls.

Reduction in Falls

The current research findings show that Bingocize® reduces the risk of falls due to a concomitant of benefits from 10-weeks of participation. The areas of improvement include the following (Crandall, Fairman & Anderson, 2015):

- all measures of muscular strength and balance were improved; and
- improvements in both upper and lower body flexibility were shown.

Research on participants who used the Bingocize® app also showed fall risk reduction in two measures (Falls et al., 2017):

- velocity of walking speeds; and
- step length.

Numerous additional studies are in progress, particularly as the pool of long-term residential participants grows from across the US to across the UK, Canada, and Eastern Europe.

Improvements in Quality of Life

Similarly, participants reported an increase in their quality of life, greatly connected to the increased socialization and joy they experienced during the Bingocize® session. Older adults are isolated much of their day, every day: "Americans ages 60 and older are alone for more than half of their daily measured time" (Livingston, 2020). Despite living in a communal center, residents of long-term facilities are not protected from experiencing social isolation or its debilitating effects (Chamberlain et al., 2020): social interaction for many geriatric persons residing in nursing homes to be six to eleven minutes per day (Thorsell et al., 2010).

The consequence of social isolation is devastating, leading to premature death and is comparable to established risk factors for mortality as obesity, substance abuse, and physical inactivity (Holt-Lunstad et al., 2015; see also Chapter 2 of this volume). Specifically, our research team (Schafer et al., 2023, p. 1136) document that Bingocize® participants report their "social isolation was significantly reduced" ($p = > 0.001$; Cohen's $d = 0.250$) during their three months, 1–2 times per week engagement (see Compliance section for the significance of attendance).

Qualitative data from Taylor and colleagues' (2020) study is also compelling. Wanda, a Bingocize® participant, notes the intergenerational engagement motivated her to attend: "Well the fellowship with the girls [peers] and the girls that come from the college [students] are always upbeat and I like that" (Taylor et al., 2020, p. 29). Joan, another participant, noted the enjoyment of the familiar game and the opportunity to meet new people: "I like to play Bingo and I like to be with people. And I enjoy being down here with my friends. And the ones that I didn't know, I know now" (Taylor et al., 2020, p. 28).

Getting long-term facility residents to attend physical activity is one feat but getting them to continue to attend is almost impossible. This is one of the exceptional aspects of Bingocize®.

Schafer and colleagues (2023) show that Bingocize® positively impacts community-dwelling older adults across four of the qualitative measures that are linked to reduction of falls and better quality of life:

1. self-reported fear of falling;
2. increased physical activity;
3. reduction of social isolation; and
4. decreased avoidance behavior.

All four results portend healthier, safer, and more content older persons living in long-term residential and those still living within their own homes. These benefits are also expected for elderly who are living in other types of communal settings, such as the incarcerated.

Compliance to Bingocize®

In part, the benefits of Bingocize® are greatly due to participants' high compliance for attendance. Schafer and colleagues found over 68% of older adults were retained over the course of the 10-week program (2023, p. 1134). This stands in stark contrast to current reports that long-term facility residents exercise less than current recommendations

(De Souto et al., 2016). A cross-sectional study by De Souto et al. (2015) showed that only 10% of nursing home residents exercised at least twice a week. Considering the robust data that attendance to physical fitness regimens has been shown to be the leading preventative measure against falls and injuries (Papalia et al., 2020), compliance findings on Bingocize® are exceptional.

Locating Bingocize®

Bingocize® is delivered live by a trained lay leader either face-to-face or using the Bingocize® web-based app. For caregivers, clinicians, or social workers seeking to help locate a local facility offering Bingocize® or enroll older persons in the web-based app, please use the Bingocize® website listed in the Resources box at the end of this chapter.

Requesting a Bingocize® License

For long-term residential activity directors, prison staff, or family members looking to initiate Bingocize® within a local facility, the application and training is straightforward. In the box below, a summary of the required steps is provided. For complete instructions, please see the Bingocize® website listed in the Resource box.

Bingocize® Licensing and Training
1. First, a license must be purchased from the Bingocize® website. Licensing fees are kept reasonable (presently, less than $500 for a two-year license) and do extend to face-to-face and online mediums, and for multiple facilities within a single county.
2. Once a license is secured, staff and/or volunteers must complete the Bingocize® asynchronous online training before conducting the Bingocize® workshop or administering the pre- and post-workshop assessments for participants. To receive Bingocize® facilitator certification, facilitators must score 80% or greater on the training competency quiz. To ensure program delivery fidelity, new facilitators are reviewed by an individual who was a current, certified Bingocize® facilitator or certified in another EBFP during the first two weeks of the training

---

workshop. The Bingocize® facilitator follows step-by-step instructions on how to lead each specific Bingocize® session, which includes strength, balance, and flexibility exercises, as well as falls prevention education (Schafer et al., 2023, p. 1131).

3. Equipment, prizes, and apparel are available for purchase through the Bingocize® website at www.bingocize.com.

Bingocize® Alternatives

If Bingocize® is unavailable in your area and the web app is not feasible, I recommend following a few of its principles when engaging with older persons in their homes, in facilities such as senior centers, clinical settings, or, even, prison settings. Combining game activities with minimal body stretches is one way to add a physical dimension to the interaction. Minimal stretches in which the person is firmly seated can safely stimulate blood flow by increasing movement. These added movements can add to the activities' enjoyment and their health benefits. A few ideas are provided in the box below.

Alternative Activities

1. Caregivers could add in hand, arm, leg stretches between plays for card games such as Rummy, Blackjack, Hearts or to games such as Dominoes, or even common board games (e.g. Sorry!™, Yahtzee™, checkers).
2. Key to adding in physical activities in environments such as home or facilities where nurses, CNAs, or other help is not readily available is to ensure the older participant is sitting and/or secure so as not to fall.
3. Participants' physical activity may not be as rigorous, but simple hand, arm, or leg movements from a sitting position still help with stiffness and circulation.
4. See the images in Figures 8.5 below, for alternative exercise movements:

Please note that any exercise regimen should be initiated after a conversation with one's physician takes place. Exercise should also be supervised to ensure the safety of all.

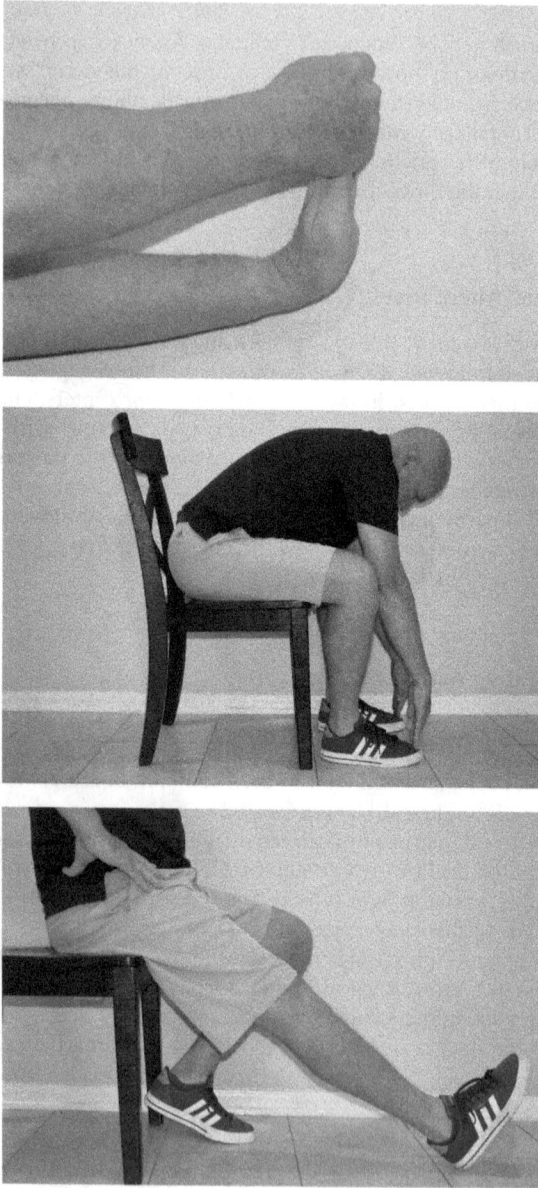

Figure 8.5 Alternative exercise images—(top to bottom) hand stretch, body
    stretch and leg stretch
Source: Rebecca Leah Johnson

Conclusion

The combination of a greatly enjoyed, well-known game with the attraction of prizes and physical movement seems the perfect solution to increasing socialization and physical fitness, developing balance, reducing fear of falls as well as actual falls and the detrimental health consequences that follow. Residents of long-term facilities and, if adopted within an easy-to-use facility, community dwelling folks are and many more could be experiencing the benefits offered by Bingocize®. I certainly look forward to this chapter helping the directors of residential activities, senior centers, rehabilitation centers, and prisons incorporate Bingocize® as part of their plans to help the populations they serve.

Questions to Consider

1. What do you think is most appealing about Bingocize® for elders?
2. Why does this form of physical activity seem to be more enjoyable than other forms of physical activity?
3. Which aspects of Bingocize® might pose the most challenges, either in planning or in execution? From a residential facility's perspective, for a caregiver, within a prison setting?
4. How might you present Bingocize® to program administrators or funding sources to secure their support to initiate Bingocize® for the elderly persons in your care?
5. What actions would you take to get participants interested in Bingocize®?

Resources

1. Bingocize® inquiries: www.wku.edu/bingocize
2. Physical guidelines for older adults:www.aafp.org/pubs/afp/issues/2010/0101/p55.html
3. The life-changing benefits of exercise after 60: www.ncoa.org/article/the-life-changing-benefits-of-exercise-after-60

References

Appeadu, M. K., & Bordoni, B. (2023). Falls and fall prevention in the elderly. www.ncbi.nlm.nih.gov/books/NBK560761/

Basiaga-Pasternak, J., & Blecharz, J. (2021). Twenty years of Studies in Sport Humanities–a look at the journal's archival issues. *Studies in Sport Humanities, 28,* 7–12.

Bertera, E. M., & Bertera, R. L. (2008). Fear of falling and activity avoidance in a national sample of older adults in the United States. *Health & Social Work, 33*(1), 54–62.

CDC. (2023). Older adult fall prevention. www.cdc.gov/falls/index.html

CDC. (2024). Older adult fall data. www.cdc.gov/falls/data/index.html

Center Stage Artists. (2024). Bingo. www.centerstageartists.com/artists/QueenofBingo/BINGOFactsHistory.doc#:~:text=There%20are%20approximately%2060%20million,play%20the%20game%20more%20often

Chamberlain, S. A., Duggleby, W., Teaster, P. B., & Estabrooks, C. A. (2020). Characteristics of socially isolated residents in long-term care: A retrospective cohort study. *Gerontology and Geriatric Medicine, 6,* 1–10.

Crandall, K. J., Fairman, C., & Anderson, J. (2015). Functional performance in older adults after a combination multicomponent exercise program and bingo game. *International Journal of Exercise Science, 8*(1), 38–48.

De Souto Barreto, P., Morley, J. E., Chodzko-Zajko, W., Pitkala, K. H., Weening-Djiksterhuis, E., Rodriguez-Mañas, L., Barbagallo, M., Rosendahl, E., Sinclair, A., Landi, F., & Network, G. G. A. R. (2016). Recommendations on physical activity and exercise for older adults living in long-term care facilities: a taskforce report. *Journal of the American Medical Directors Association, 17*(5), 381–392.

De Souto, B. P., Demougeot, L., Vellas, B., & Rolland, Y. (2015). How much exercise are older adults living in nursing homes doing in daily life? A cross-sectional study. *Journal of Sports Science, 33*(2), 116–124.

Dispennette, A. K., Schafer, M. A., Shake, M., Clark, B., Macy, G. B., Vanover, S., & Crandall, K. J. (2019). Effects of a game-centered health promotion program on fall risk, health knowledge, and quality of life in community-dwelling older adults. *International Journal of Exercise Science, 12*(4), 1149.

Falls, D. G., Crandall, K. J., Shake, M., & Arnett, S. (2017). Efficacy of a mobile application for improving gait performance in community-dwelling older adults. Master's thesis, Western Kentucky University.

Holt-Lunstad J., Smith, T. B., Baker, M., Harris, T., & Stephenson, D. (2015). Loneliness and social isolation as risk factors for mortality: A meta-analytic review. *Perspectives on Psychological Science, 10*(2), 227–237.

Kelly, M., Clarke, B., Ghiara, V., Russo, F., Bockting, C., Boniolo, G., Canali, S., Conforti, M., Dedef, C., Frezza, G., & Vineiss, P. (2019). Time to care: Why the humanities and the social sciences belong in the science of health. *BMJ Open, 9*:e030286. https://doi.org/10.1136/bmjopen-2019-030286

Komisar, V., Dojnov, A., Yang, Y., Shishov, N., Chong, H., Yu, Y., Bercovitz, I., Cusimano, M. D., Becker, C., Mackey, D. C., & Robinovitch, S. N. (2022). Injuries from falls by older adults in long-term care captured on video: Prevalence of impacts and injuries to body parts. *BMC Geriatrics*, 22(1), 343. https://doi.org/10.1186/s12877-022-03041-3.

Livingston, G. (2020). On average, older adults spend over half their waking hours alone. *Pew Research Center*. www.pewresearch.org/fact-tank/2019/07/03/on-average-older-adults-spend-over-half-their-waking-hours-alone/

Marks, R., Allegrante, J. P., MacKenzie, C. R., & Lane, J. M. (2003). Hip fractures among the elderly: causes, consequences and control. *Ageing Research Reviews*, 2(1), 57–93.

National Bingo Game. (2024). Facts. www.nationalbingo.co.uk/interesting-facts#:~:text=Bingo%20originated%20in%20Italy%20and,a%20fair%20in%20Jacksonville%20Georgia

Oliver, D., Papaioannou, A., Giangregorio, L., Thabane, L., Reizgys, K., & Foster, G. (2008). A systematic review and meta-analysis of studies using the STRATIFY tool for prediction of falls in hospital patients: how well does it work?. *Age and Ageing*, 37(6), 621–627.

Papalia, G. F., Papalia, R., Diaz Balzani, L. A., Torre, G., Zampogna, B., Vasta, S., Fossati, C., Alifano, A.M., & Denaro, V. (2020). The effects of physical exercise on balance and prevention of falls in older people: A systematic review and meta-analysis. *Journal of Clinical Medicine*, 9(8), 2595.

Peel, N. M., Alapatt, L. J., Jones, L. V., & Hubbard, R. E. (2019). The association between gait speed and cognitive status in community-dwelling older people: a systematic review and meta-analysis. *The Journals of Gerontology: Series A*, 74(6), 943–948.

Schafer, M. A., Upright, P., Michalik, J., & Crandall, K. J. (2023). Impact of 10-week evidence–based falls prevention program on outcomes related to falls risk in community-dwelling older adults. *International Journal of Exercise Science*, 16(7), 1131–1141.

Soulé, B., Marchant, G., & Verchère, R. (2022). Sport and fitness app uses: A review of humanities and social science perspectives. *European Journal for Sport and Society*, 19(2), 170–189.

Tak, S. H., Kedia, S., Tongumpun, T. M., & Hong, S. H. (2015). Activity engagement: Perspectives from nursing home residents with dementia. *Educational Gerontology*, 41(3), 182–192.

Taylor, J., Piatt, J., Stanojevic, C., Crandall, K. J., & C-EP, A. C. S. M. (2020). Bingocize® beyond the numbers: Motivations and perceptions of a multicomponent health promotion program among older adults living in long-term care. *American Journal of Recreation Therapy*, 19(1), 23–34.

Thorsell, K. B. E., Nordström, B. M., Fagerström, L., & Sivberg, B. V. (2010). Time in care for older people living in nursing homes, *Nursing Research and Practice*, https://doi.org/10.1155/2010/148435

9 Learning Together

Intergenerational Activities for Residential Centers

Trini Stickle, Jessica L. Folk and Cameron Fontes

Objectives

By the end of this chapter:

1. You are expected to better understand the effect of three different activities designed to increase intergenerational engagement between young adults and older persons: collaborative storytelling, postcard exchanges, and creating video-recorded instructional media.
2. You should be able to conduct each activity using the materials and steps provided.
3. You should be able to instruct others in conducting these activities and/or generate similar activities to do or share.
4. You should be able to provide a rationale for such activities based on the theoretical and empirical support provided in this chapter.

Introduction

As described in chapter two and emphasized throughout this book, the most pressing concerns of and for our elderly citizens are isolation, loneliness and the cascade of both physical and mental deterioration that follow from such living conditions. To help address these issues as members within the academic community, we participated in the collegiate, extra-curricular student group Companions of Respected Elders (CORE) whose mission was to provide for intergenerational interaction. Stickle and Folk present their experiences as advisors, and Fontes presents his reflections as CORE's co-president and his experiences as a group member. The group's goals and activities illustrate one way the next generation can learn from and provide companionship to members of our older generation. This student group initially began as a part

DOI: 10.4324/9781003359463-11

of a geriatric-focused certificate program with the goal of providing an avenue for college students, largely in health care majors, to better understand health issues and the milieu of aging. As members interacted with elderly living in residential centers, these experiences afforded students better communication skills essential for their future professions. CORE experienced a short period of inactivity and dormant status due to the loss of our institute's geriatric program. When it was reinstituted, what evolved was something with less of a professional development and more of a person-centered focus, more equitably beneficial for all participants. In practice, during these Saturday meetings, what emerged were relationships *between* the college students and the elderly residents. Students and the residents of local nursing homes grew together as companions as roles were shared and equally respected, and the group's name Companions of Respected Elders truly manifested. In this chapter, we chronicle CORE's development through descriptions of and reflections on three activities while offering guidance for current students and leaders to facilitate similar activities: Co-creating Moments, Continuing Conversations through Correspondence, and Writing for Longevity. Additionally, we are hopeful the theoretical and empirical support and examples will lead our readers to create additional activities that will create inclusive opportunities for intergenerational engagement.

Context

When Folk and Stickle became involved as faculty advisors to CORE, the mission focused on professional communication; we, instead, emphasized the positive, social implications for all the participants involved in these intergenerational interactions. To better facilitate those goals, both CORE faculty advisors and students were trained through the communication methods of TimeSlips©, a non-profit organization that works to innervate the lives of elderly persons through evidenced-based, collaborative storytelling (more on TimeSlips© provided in the Resources box of this chapter). The training consists of perfecting listening and questioning skills that have been shown to foster meaningful interactions for elderly participants and their co-participants (Bahlke, Pericolosi & Lehman, 2010). Timeslips© techniques present best practices in communicating with persons experiencing loss of memory, impaired hearing and other common aging issues (Vigliotti, Chinchilli & George, 2017). As new student members joined, they were asked to complete the TimeSlips© training before they participated in visits to residential centers. The purpose of the TimeSlips training is to encourage and foster the skills for intergenerational engagement, instill positive attitudes on aging, and to increase the likelihood of volunteer activities throughout young persons' lives by establishing the practice and motivation during the college years (Heuer, 2020; Fritsch et al., 2009). These hopeful, socially positive outcomes are, and continue to be, borne out by empirical findings.

As advisors to CORE, we purposefully empowered our student members to take charge of the group's operations, providing necessary support but encouraging student autonomy. Once CORE members achieved the required training through TimeSlips©, members were tasked with contacting and coordinating engagements with local residential center activity directors, ensuring compliance with the procedures to engage in activities within these centers, scheduling events and conducting storytelling activities at the centers (a step-by-step summary follows in section Activity 1). Once recurring activities were established, CORE members augmented story-telling activities with visits for holiday-themed craft projects (e.g., Christmas, Hanukkah, Valentine's Day) as well as visits for game nights.

When COVID-19 entered the United States in spring of 2020, creating a lethal hazard for our elderly population (see chapter 2 for a thorough description), students were unable to meet with residents for face-to-face activities due to the strict and necessary safety precautions initiated. In response, CORE members began a postcard campaign, initially using the Beautiful Question postcards acquired freely through TimeSlips© (see the Resources box in this chapter), later adding other types of correspondence. Space was left available on the Beautiful Question postcards for residents who were able and willing to respond, and a small number of residents did so, sending back their annotated cards through a CORE member who worked as a certified nurse attendant (CNA) at one of the residential facilities. As of the writing of these chapters, the postcard/card practices remain active, allowing continued, albeit mediated, interaction but sustained contact with residents (a step-by-step summary follows in section Activity 2). Lastly, in the summer of 2020, CORE members created a recorded writing workshop for members of a local seniors' group facilitated by a public library (the details follow in the section Activity 3). We believe these interactions have helped mitigate the consequential isolation and loneliness of aging, exacerbated by the COVID-19 pandemic, but which is, too often, the daily, taxing experience of our elderly population, both those living within and outside of residential facilities. Without our own empirical studies on this small sample of activities and participants, we draw support for this claim from the findings on the TimeSlips© program as well as from tangential findings on intergenerational interactions and service-learning research focused on interactions between young adults and older generations. Compiled within their meta-analysis, Eyler and colleagues (2001) report the effects of service learning for college students, faculty, the institutions and communities. Consistent with Eyler's et al. (2001) findings, we observed student growth in areas such a sense of personal efficacy, personal identity, spiritual growth and moral development, in leadership and communication skills, and a reduction in age or aging bias. As faculty, we concur with the findings of increased satisfaction with our student interactions, a renewed sense of research and/or creative activities, and a personal increase in our volunteer commitment. We illustrate these observations in the reflections posted below each activity.

Despite the unusual circumstances that led to the distanced interactions of the later activities, the authors advocate that both in-person and distanced interactions are helpful for elderly persons in residential centers, home care and other populations who experience increased isolation as a result of incarceration, a decline in socioeconomic status or poverty, emigration and/or other factors. We now present step-by-step guidance for participating in the three CORE activities—storytelling, postcard correspondence, video workshops—and provide corresponding lists of needed materials. After the activities are described, we present reflections of our experiences.

Activity 1 Summary: Co-creating Moments (Stories, Crafts, Games)

We begin with the primary and focused activity of CORE, collaborative storytelling. For this activity, we followed the guidance and training provided by TimeSlips©. We encourage interested readers to consult its website and complete the training to ensure constructing questions and issuing encouragement to the elderly participants is done using techniques designed to reduce stress and maximize the collaborative effects of storytelling. Key to the storytelling activities conducted with elders is the emphasis that the stories are not meant to rely on actual, personal memories. One strength of this collaborative activity is that the details of setting, characters, action (plot) arise from easily accessible and context-free participant contributions. Difficulties and deficits in memory retrieval are ameliorated by following this approach, making the cooperative process interactional, engaging, enjoyable and stress-free. We present the basic items needed and the generic steps to follow.

Materials

1. A means of presenting visual notes on the stories created—a shared Word document, Google Doc, or other note-taking software. An easel with a large pad of paper works well.
2. Markers (if the story is created on a large pad of paper).
3. Images and objects that serve to prompt the participants to generate ideas for the setting, the characters and the plot.

Steps to Activity

1. The residents of health care facilities gather in an open area such as the cafeteria or activities room.
2. The facilitators introduce themselves and the activity.
3. To begin the creative process, a prompt is introduced. The prompt is usually a visual of some sort like a photograph, a painting, an online or print illustration. A tangible item works just as well when conducting the activity in-person at a facility. These items should not be personal to the participants (e.g., a photo of a family member), as this may put pressure on them to recall particular experiences or memories surrounding the object.
4. The residents are invited to respond to the prompt through free-association—whatever comes to mind from the image or object and whatever details are generated from the interaction amongst the participants, without the stress of retrieving personal memories or factual details. Key is that all contributions are recognized as helpful in the generation of the story.
5. A facilitator records the suggestions. We found that a large pad of paper and an easel worked well for the participants to see the process and have the visual of the words present.
6. From the words and phrases, a facilitator reiterates the suggestions and encourages the participants to create a story from them. This process is completed one sentence at a time as contributed from and negotiated among the different participants.
7. No rules are imposed for how the story "should" develop, rather, this activity is less about creating a coherent narrative and more about allowing for a means of personal expression amongst the residents and participants where all ideas are honored.
8. The facilitator synthesizes the ideas and retells the story to the group based on the participants' suggestions, and, later, transcribes the sentence-to-sentence story.

Optional: The facilitators may transcribe the completed story, editing for coherence, while still maintaining the intended storyline, add additional images and create a paper copy to share with the residents upon the next visit. Additionally, the residents' stories may be posted on a bulletin board at the entrance of the facility/home, or stories created over the course of the year may be shared with family and friends via a digital presentation such as PowerPoint®, a PDF or a printed, bound collection.

Craft and game activities followed as relationships between CORE student members, residents and staff afforded additional visits.

Reflection

Having occasionally attended the storytelling activities with the CORE student members, our experience as the faculty advisors was, first, a unified sense of hope for a society too often segregated by age. Hope became joy as we watched the residential participants and CORE students working together, laughing, gasping in "shock," or wincing in fear as they animated the characters of the unfolding story as each filled with details of time and place—often built from memories—and that ultimately came together with simple plots turning into a completed narrative. Residents of the facility who were in wheelchairs moved closer to the facilitators, studying the prompt, to share their details. Others shared their contributions loudly or enlisted another CORE member to share, especially if unable to raise to an audible level due to oxygen tubes or other such medical apparatus.

Often, after the sessions, as CORE members circulated the room to say their goodbyes, hands would reach out for a gentle touch, a pat, a lingering hold and a few additional words to keep the students near for a few minutes more. Our reflections will always include the sense of witnessing something bigger than just a visit to a residential center, something grander than the creation of a simple story.

Activity 2 Summary: Continuing Conversations through Correspondence

We began with a simple goal of letting our residential companions know that we were still thinking of them and that we wished to continue our conversations despite the inability to visit them face to face. First, CORE members wrote out simple notes using the Beautiful Question postcards obtained from TimeSlips© and dropped them off at residential centers that we had been regularly visiting. One of the CORE members who worked as a CNA at another nursing home brought a stack to her residents, and she was also able to collect the responses added by the residents, themselves, or by way of family members or aids.

Since we are a university extracurricular club, word of our postcard campaign made its rounds through campus. As a result, one of the composition instructors asked whether his first-year students could contribute postcards as part of a unit on writing for different registers (i.e., audiences), a class that also included an option for such a service-learning activity. CORE members with the help of current students enrolled in the (above) instructor's composition classes continue to write out post-cards and other types of cards each semester. A CORE member or a faculty advisor couriered the stacks of correspondence to various residential facilities, leaving the cards with the centers' activities directors who then provided the means for distribution.

Materials

1. Postcards, other cards, handcrafted notes, or even notecards (e.g., 3 × 5 cards) (see also TimeSlips© for Beautiful Question postcard requests);
2. A connection within residential centers such as their activities directors or other staff members. (This is easily facilitated by a phone call.)

Steps to Activity

1. Distribute the postcards or other cards to volunteers.
2. Set a date, time and place to collect completed cards.
3. Designate a person to drop off stacks of completed cards to facilities.
4. If the staff at a given residential center plans to facilitate responses by the residential participants, negotiate a day and time for pick up.

This activity is such a simple one that it may seem wholly unnecessary to write out needed materials and procedural steps to include in a work such as this, but we believe the benefits of this activity outweigh its simplicity, and while the positive outcomes of such activities are understudied, a few studies are worth noting. Binnie's 2019 study on the effects of her intergenerational correspondence program *Writing Back* (2014–2018) is a first. She states that after a fifty-study review of intergenerational activities designed to alleviate loneliness in the elderly and/or student populations, "none of the interventions involved letter writing between different age groups" (p. 62), despite numerous studies on the positive effects of correspondence, in general that show "physical and mental benefits across diverse samples" (Pennebaker & Seagal, 1999, p. 1252). These include "improve[d] well-being and significantly decrease[d] levels of depressive symptoms" (Toepfer et al.,

2012, p. 198) as well as reductions in incidences of self-harm (Harris, 2002, p. 2). Binnie's study reports on the intergenerational correspondence between elderly and college participants writing about their experiences of loneliness as a writing intervention to mitigate loneliness and its negative consequences. Using the lens of narrative inquiry—the accounts as found in the letters themselves—augmented with questionnaire data provided by the participants. Binnie reports that "89 per cent of students ($n = 19$) and 91 percent of older participants ($n = 34$) agreed that writing to their pen pal had a positive effect on their mental well-being" (2019, p. 69); students reported that the activity helped keeping their "brains working" as the elderly participants similarly reported the correspondence worked to "hone our skills of communication and keep our brain active" (Binnie, 2019, p. 70). Sentiments on the effects of receiving and writing letters regarding the experience of loneliness are summed by Binnie's older respondent Jane: "I live alone and it is really nice to receive a letter and take time to write back about what I have been doing or what I have done in the past" and her college-age respondent Emily:

> Letters and letter writing seem like a great way to combat loneliness both for students and the older generation . . . it seems therapeutic to me as well and distracts you from problems and stresses of everyday life. It is something to look forward to!
>
> (Binnie, 2019, p. 70)

We conjecture that our postcard campaign serves its writers and recipients equally well, and we offer the below reflection as one, small window of one such continuing, positive effect.

Reflection

In personal correspondence with the instructor who continues to involve his first-year composition students in the CORE postcard/card campaign, he noted:

> I have always encouraged my English foundations classes to participate in writing projects outside of the classroom to underscore the importance of using their voice to make a difference in the community-at-large. The CORE postcard sharing project has been an extremely popular activity, probably the most popular of all the community outreach opportunities I give them. Not only do the students eagerly commit themselves to the endeavor during the semester, the postcard project makes a lasting impact as well.

Just a few weeks ago, a student told me that over the previous weekend, she had been inspired by her participation in the CORE postcards last semester to handwrite fifty-four Valentines for the residents of the retirement center in which her grandmother had passed away.

(Jon Meyers, WKU English instructor)

Activity 3 Summary: Writing for Longevity, a Recorded Workshop

At the request of a local public library, CORE members created a recorded activity that could be shared with a senior group whose monthly meetings had been upended with the lockdowns caused by COVID-19. Relying heavily on our residential storytelling experiences and playing on the strengths of our screenwriter (Folk) and our CORE co-president's (Fontes) creative writing talents along with the technical and narrative skills of both CORE's co-president (Samantha Eaton) and co-advisor (Stickle), we agreed to create the three-part writing workshop: *Writing for Longevity*. Adding to our decision were everyone's experience of increased limited interactions that led to hours alone with thoughts and memories. We focused our help on prompts that would best lead to short autobiographical sketches, memoirs, or creative pieces appropriate for sharing with their friends and families. Our goals were to provide easy-to-follow videos that generated memories allowing direct translation to prose or ideas into plots; a how-to guide for word processing, and various methods by which they could distribute their productions, or, quite simply, step-by-step directions on how to get their stories into the hands and hearts of others. Of the three activities, this may be the most technically challenging for others to reproduce; however, with the aid of cellphone video capture, we expect those challenges are greatly overcome. Additionally, while we created a workshop to fit our talent pool, we encourage readers to select a skill or activity they could "teach" through their own video workshop or to find ways to entertain their viewers. Skill-development workshops span the gamut of possibilities from other creative outlets within the arts, such as painting; crafts; technical abilities such as how to better make use of the features of one's cellular phone or computer; or providing a video aid for negotiating different health care or other facilities in the local area. Again, these suggestions merely introduce the potential for providing our elderly and their caregivers information when faced with the isolating effects of being home or facility bound.

Materials

1. A means to record in an mp4 or .mov format: phone, computer or tablet with a webcam, video camera. If describing or demonstrating an activity, a cell phone video capturing application would work fine. If using the aid of documents, then some form of a computer software program would work best: Quicktime®, Zoom®, PowerPoint® narrated slideshow, Screencastify®, or any number of other such programs.
2. A cloud housing storage system to share the links to the recordings with the intended group.
3. A working script to keep the presenter(s) on task and within time.

Steps to Activity

1. Create a working script for the skill you wish to share.
2. Gather or create the materials needed to share with your group as you record.
3. Record the presentation. If possible, choose a transcription or closed caption option that will record a text version of the talk for hearing-impaired elders. Alternatively, receivers of the recorded presentation may be able to select a playback feature for live-transcription or closed captioning. When working with a community group or residential center, these types of options should be explored.
4. Depending on the skill level of the creator(s), editing of the video may be possible.
5. Save the recorded presentation, so the link to that presentation can be easily shared with the intended population. Most residential centers could easily show video presentations with an internet connection and a monitor with speakers.

Reflection

When I reflect on my visits to care facilities as a CORE member (Fontes), I'm grateful not only for how they provided me real-life inspiration for my work as a creative writer, but most of all for how they reinforced my suspicion that the fear of growing older is based largely in myth, and that with age doesn't just come a limiting but also a broadening of opportunities and new beginnings. I could have framed my interactions with the elders I met with sadness because of their health issues or their proximity to the end of life; instead, I took their stories, memories and creative ideas as a preview of how life can be well-lived to its end. The lasting impact of these interactions reminds me now to reach out to those closest to me who accept me as I am and who build me up when times get hard—and encourages me to do the same for them. Life consists of relationships, and it is our connections to each other that will save us when times get hard. From my CORE experiences, I am reminded I can and should help foster connections between elders and other members of my community as I forge my own path in the world. As members of communities local and global, our personal drive for success and purpose need not isolate us from others as we work ever harder to find what we're looking for, as we overcome barriers of time and distance and of generational differences during all of life's stages.

Post-COVID CORE Update

Full engagement for both faculty and students proved to be slow for several academic semesters after the institutional COVID-19 protocols were relaxed and finally disbanded. Both a health-motivated fear and a loss of sociability infiltrated many folks' daily lives post-pandemic. For CORE, we slowly rebuilt and reorganized. Between fall of 2020 and spring of 2021, I (Stickle) began the academic year with one CORE member, Hannah Lanham, a communication disorders major. Hannah increased student awareness of the isolation experienced by persons in nursing homes; she tabled for CORE around campus; she shared the goals of CORE with fellow health and humanities majors, alike. She increased student interest in CORE, and our numbers began to grow. The new CORE cohort struggled to engage with persons living in residential centers due to the centers continued restrictions. Yet, CORE members continued a robust letter correspondence campaign, dropping off stacks of notes to various residential centers along with flowers and holiday crafts to brighten the residents' days and to reassure them that this body of undergraduate students cared about them. CORE membership grew to eight students. By fall 2022, CORE members were allowed back into the residential centers, and CORE, now with its largest membership of any time (14 members), had resumed in-person visits that include collaborative storytelling, crafts and conversations. In the academic year 2022/23, CORE membership grew to 21 students, who visited residential centers 16 times. CORE continues to be a growing and strong student group today.

Conclusion

As isolation negatively affects the mental and physical well-being of all of us, we offer these activities as well as the many others inspired by them as conduits to engage with the older persons, the persons with dementia, and their caregivers in our communities. We are hopeful that our presentation of CORE's activities, as well as the many other activities presented in this collection, encourages our readers to find ways to connect with members of our older population or to begin an intergenerational network with them as we strive for better individual and collective health and well-being. We also believe that each of us as part of this university-sponsored club witnessed an intergenerational connectedness that promises our ability to survive and thrive amid social, political and health crises together.

Questions to Consider

1. If you were to conduct each of the activities, what do you anticipate will require the most preparation, and what are the steps of your plan to ensure the most positive experience for each?
2. If you had to provide a rationale for one of the activities in order to garner funding for such a club or for the activities illustrated here, what evidence or theoretical support would you use?
3. If you were to alter one of the activities, what would you change and why?

Resources

1. TimeSlips©: www.timeslips.org
2. Beautiful Questions. TimeSlips©: www.timeslips.org/resources/creativity-center
3. Campaign to End Loneliness: www.campaigntoendloneliness.org
4. The Silver Line: www.thesilverline.org.uk

References

Bahlke, L., Pericolosi, S., & Lehman, M. (2010). Use of TimeSlips to improve communication in persons with moderate–late stage dementia. *Journal of Aging, Humanities, and the Arts, 4*(4), 390–405.

Binnie, G. (2019). Loneliness and the letter: Co-developing cross-generational letter writing with higher education students and older people. *Research for All, 3*(1), 59–73. https://doi.org/10.18546/RFA.03.1.06

Eyler, J., Giles, D. E. Jr., Stenson, C. M., & Gray, C. J. (2001). At a glance: What we know about the effects of service-learning on college students, faculty, institutions and communities, 1993–2000. http://digitalcommons.unomaha.edu/slcehighered/139

Fritsch, T., Kwak, J., Grant, S., Lang, J., Montgomery, R. R., & Basting, A. D. (2009). Impact of TimeSlips, a creative expression intervention program, on nursing home residents with dementia and their caregivers, *The Gerontologist, 49*(1), 117–127. https://doi.org/10.1093/geront/gnp008

Harris, J. (2002) The correspondence method as a data-gathering technique in qualitative enquiry. *International Journal of Qualitative Methods, 1*(4), 1–9.

Heuer, S. (2020). The Impact of TimeSlips on undergraduate students in service learning with older adults. *Perspectives of the ASHA Special Interest Groups, 6*(1), 122–129.

Pennebaker, J. W., & Seagal, J. D. (1999). Forming a story: The health benefits of narrative. *Journal of Clinical Psychology, 55*(10), 1243–1254.

Toepfer, S. M., Cichy, K., & Peters, P. (2012). Letters of gratitude: Further evidence for author benefits. *Journal of Happiness Studies, 13*(1), 187–201.

Vigliotti, A. A., Chinchilli, V. M., & George, D. R. (2017). Enhancing quality of life and caregiver interactions for persons with dementia using TimeSlips group storytelling: A 6-month longitudinal study. *The American Journal of Geriatric Psychiatry: Official Journal of the American Association for Geriatric Psychiatry, 26*(4), 507–508.

10 Who Can I Talk to When Nobody's Here with Me?

Meredith Troutman-Jordan,
Margaret Maclagan and Boyd H. Davis

Objectives

By the end of this chapter:

1. You will better understand the effects of using robotic (i.e., animatronic) pets as companions for older persons and persons diagnosed with memory issues.
2. You will be able to facilitate the 'adoption' of robotic pets by older persons.
3. You will be able to advocate for the implementation of a robotic pet companion program within your facility based on the empirical and qualitative data provided in this chapter.
4. You will be able to demonstrate the benefits of the robot pet for starting conversations.

Introduction

The issue of pervasive loneliness and its health consequences for the older population, including those suffering from cognitive difficulties, has been core to this collection. The social aspects of care are an essential motivation for our focus within geriatric undergraduate and graduate studies, whether the courses are within nursing or other clinical programs, social work, or health care management. Health humanities provides us an inroad for treating patients or long-term residents with dignity, ensuring their basic human needs are met and respected while ameliorating symptoms of illnesses.

The need for companionship is essential to humanity. We need to share a space with others and in that space have conversations, empathize, express care, share memories and make new memories. The importance of conversation as a human need aligns with the theoretical perspective within Cognitive Pragmatics (e.g., Bosco & Tirassa, 2022)

DOI: 10.4324/9781003359463-12

and magnifies the difficulties members of our aging population face when such human contact and conversation become minimally available to them. Yet, we are aware of this reality: friends, family members, formal and informal caregivers simply cannot always be available to serve as companions to older persons, particularly those with dementia. Consequently, on most days, many may be deprived of this simple, basic need to feel connected (Davis et al., 2021).

One solution for many older people has been to assign service animals to them. This draws on the role pets play in the home to provide emotional well-being, especially for persons at risk of social isolation (Beck & Katcher, 1996). Research has documented the positive effects these four-legged companions provide: ameliorating loneliness, reducing depression and anxiety, and increasing verbal output (cf. Ambrosi et al., 2019; review by Chang et al., 2021). However, not all residential arrangements allow live animal companions and not all older persons can provide the care that a live animal requires. In this chapter, we offer our findings on the next best solution, robotic or animatronic pets.

Animatronic pets such as the Joy for All™ provide comfort and connection for persons living with dementia and can be successful in any living situation. In this chapter, we report observations after introducing a robotic pet to an older person living with dementia, provide several conversation starters derived from our observations of older persons interacting by themselves with robotic pets, and interacting with their pets and caregivers. This work has also facilitated experiential learning opportunities, research course topics and workshops that address these specific companion solutions (Troutman-Jordan, 2021). The authors share suggestions for ways to implement these practices for personal and/or institutional care.

Background

Our goal is to advance empirically supported activities that keep aging persons—including older persons living with dementia—engaged with others and the world around them. Key to this process is the amelioration of loneliness and isolation which has been shown to advance physical and cognitive decline and expedite mortality (see Chapter 2). Conversational interaction is central to our joint concerns as it affords older adults a means of maintaining and expressing oneself (Matsumoto, 2011, 2019). Studies on conversational interaction for persons living with dementia demonstrate the power of conversation in anchoring their identities, maintaining their personhood and reinforcing their will to live. This can be seen in current research as well as in a sample of earlier studies (e.g., Davis, 2005; Guendouzi & Müller, 2006; Hamilton, 1994; Ramanathan, 1997; Ryan et al., 2005). A key aid to conversation engagement for people experiencing cognitive issues is "an object present here and now," as first noted in Hamilton's work (2011) and continued in others (e.g., Isaac & Hamilton, 2020; Stickle, 2023). Such a focus obviates the need for remembering specific facts or details and allows all participants equal access to the topic at hand, reducing the vocabulary needed for the talk. The stress of producing language within the conversation is thus reduced. Objects of art, other physical items present in the visual sphere and service animals (Kirk et al., 2019) have served in the role of conversation topic. We focus here on the role and advantages that a robotic pet provides when it serves as a potential focus for conversation.

AI, Animatronics and Geriatric Care

The growing industry of robotics for elder care has arisen to meet several challenges. Improvements in quality of life is foremost: the need to maximize older persons' independence (Van Assche et al., 2022); a means to reduce loneliness (Hudson et al., 2020); and respite time to help prevent caregiver burnout (Santhanajaraj et al., 2021).

Despite these and other therapeutic benefits, critics have expressed concern that animatronic pets could potentially cause confusion between reality and illusion. Some voice concerns that providing a robotic pet could be perceived as deception, consequently, leading to the infantilization of persons living with dementia (Vercelli et al., 2017). Similarly, Coghlan and colleagues argue such practice could be a threat to one's sense of autonomy and dignity (2021).

The purpose of our initial study on the specific use of robotic pets in dementia care was to better determine whether their use served the community of persons living with dementia in positive ways or did their use evoke negative consequences. We evaluated these determinations by interviewing caregivers about their perceptions of animatronic pets as companions for the persons living with dementia and their perceptions of the effects such simulated pets had on persons within their care.

Context

Our study arose in a special topics graduate gerontology course focused on the exploration of robotic pets in dementia care. The course employed an experiential learning activity that required graduate students to participate in the collection of data from families who received a robotic pet. Graduate students completed research training (i.e., CITI training) and interview methodology prior to data collection. Families were selected through snowball sampling:[1] graduate students within the course invited known families caring for persons living with dementia to participate. Nine families agreed to participate in the study. A Joy for All™ cat or dog was provided to each family through university funding for special topics courses. Families selected their pet based on comments made by their care recipients, suggesting preferences for a cat or a dog keyed to prior experiences. Families kept the pet at the end of the observation period. The Joy for All™ pets were chosen because of their relatively low cost. (Present cost of these specific robotic pets averages between one hundred and twenty-five to one hundred and fifty dollars each.)[2]

Observations and interviews with the caregivers were conducted in the participants' homes or a preferred neutral location selected by a family. Observations included the interactions between the person living with dementia and their "cat" or "dog"; interview questions captured the caregivers' perceptions of the effects the robotic pet had on the person living with dementia and on the overall caregiving process. The interview questions are located in the Appendix. Interviews varied in duration, but they tended to last 10–15 minutes. All interviews were audio-recorded and transcribed verbatim.

Findings and Applications

From our analyses of the observations and interview data, five themes emerged on the usefulness of a Joy for All™ pet as a companion and aid in the care of persons living with dementia. Overall, views of the caregivers were positive, describing various ways the robotic pets benefitted the persons living with dementia, with only a few limitations identified. A discussion of themes is shared below. Following the findings, we provide guidance for the introduction and implementation of a robotic pet into the care of a person living with dementia.

Theme 1: Someone to Talk to

Overwhelmingly, these pets proved to be welcomed, "listening companions," something non-judgmental to talk to for each of their "owners." The caregivers reported that persons living with dementia typically initiated conversations with the pets without inhibitions. These reports stand in contrast to the reported hesitations or apprehensions about being understood during person-to-person interactions (e.g., Clare & Shakespeare, 2004). Our research shows persons living with dementia felt free to talk to their pets without worrying about their pets' behavior or response to them. Each caregiver reported impressions of the pets' therapeutic benefits. We report a sampling of those impressions.

First, the robotic pets provided an incentive to speak even when communications with other humans had decreased or stopped altogether. One daughter stated that her mother:

> [p]retty much stopped communicating with us, other than when we would ask her a question, she responded, but she always communicated with the robotic animals. It was like she was more social with them than she was with people.

The pets gave persons living with dementia motivation for their own care. A long-term care therapist commented that her patient would express encouragement and motivate her own progress through her pet:

> She will often talk to Dash while completing therapy in which she says things like "Come on, Dash, we can do it," or "Dash, let's try to walk outside today it is a beautiful day." Prior to Dash, she was never interested in engaging in physical therapy outside of her daughter's house.

The therapist noticed similar reactions in other patients who had been given a robotic pet:

> This lady rarely smiled and often was not motivated or fully focused during physical therapy. We meet twice a week for physical therapy, and the change in her mood, speech, and behavior has been measurable. Prior to Dash some visits she would not be dressed and motivating her to even get out of bed, at times, it was next to impossible. She appears to be both motivated and enthusiastic about both life and physical therapy.

Persons living with dementia were also reported to find new joy in daily life as expressed through their conversations with their pet. One woman shared her mother's daily interactions with her pet:

> My mother talks to Dash daily, either telling him how cute he is or asking Dash if he is ready to take a nap with her. She treats Dash like a member of the family which works for me because Dash, her Joy for All™ pet, seems to consistently make her smile. Dash simply does no wrong.

For persons living with dementia, the pets were something they could relate to through conversations which often focused on set routines and activities, perhaps affording a sense of consistency and normalcy.

Several caregivers described the comfort their person living with dementia derived from the constancy of the pet and their sense of relatedness to it. The pets also gave rise to increased verbal output in ways that other humans did not and replaced negative emotions with positive ones. For example, one woman shared:

> Mom seems to be more vocal these days as prior to her Joy for All™ pet Dash, she stayed very quiet and, in many ways, [was] depressed and reserved. She still has days in which she can be moody, but she seems to feel a sense of comfort, and calmness while holding or even sleeping with Dash . . . Social communication and skills have improved as she appears to introduce her new companion instead of sitting silently and not participating or engaging while in family and church engagements.

Even when increased conversations with pets did not lead to increased conversations with others, family members reported hearing the talk between their relatives and their pet. A daughter said of her father, "I have not noticed any difference in Dad's speech, just that he talks to 'Boots' a lot." This last comment is particularly important as it reminds us that providing a robotic pet for persons under care may not open conversation pathways with other humans. Yet, the findings are hopeful for families or institutions looking for a relatively inexpensive means to bring comfort and joy to persons living with dementia.

Theme 2: Continuous Love, Companionship

The presence of the robotic pet often initiated a new and deeper relationship for the person living with dementia. Caregivers described how the robotic pet became more than an object; instead, caregivers believed their family members saw the pet as a loyal friend and companion. Caregivers provided detailed descriptions that illustrated feelings of unconditional, continuous love and companionship experienced by the person living with dementia. As one daughter commented:

> [W]ell, her behavior changed. Just as soon as you turned it on because a big smile would come on her face. And, other than that, she didn't smile that much. So, yes, her behavior changed then, and, like I said, she talked to the robotic pets more than she talked to people. So as far as the communication was, I mean, she used to talk to her real dogs also in place of people before the robotic pets, but, that's you know, of course (pause) really, it really helped her emotionally.

The daughter also shared how the pet worked to reduce her mother's frustration because she confused her caregiver daughter with her sister:

> [S]he always thought I was her sister so she and her and her sister didn't get along very well, so she was always, you know (pause) *at* me more than anybody else, and if I handed her that pet, and you know, she, she was content. And, and she wasn't, and she wasn't fussing at me anymore.

Theme 3: Mental Health Benefits

For some persons living with dementia, the pets provided mental health benefits and initiated new, hopeful perspectives regarding their own personal lives. One caregiver explained:

> Before she received her Joy for All™ pet Mom went through a battle with depression. In the time of a little over a year and a half prior to receiving Dash she was not only a widow, [but also] lost her youngest son, broke her hip, was diagnosed with dementia, and had to sell everything she ever knew. (pause) She stopped her social activities that she loved when she also moved, such as going to church, and became isolated. When you brought her Joy for All™ pet, her dog, she smiles more, socializes more, and stays involved in church activities. (pause) Dash has made a major difference in her mood. She used to get frustrated some days when she couldn't remember things, and now she appears to stay calm if she has Dash by her side.

Most caregiver participants shared specific examples of how the pets provided a continuous source of love that improved mood and behavior. One caregiver described poignantly the magnitude of the pet's significance for the mental health of her brother:

> I can tell his mood has changed a lot for the better. He is bipolar and has extremely bad depression that has made him suicidal a couple of times. My brother was in Vietnam, and it was not good for him. (pause) I see a difference in his mood and personality since he got his new friend. He bragged about his new pet and thought it was cool. He kept it in his lap or the bed when he laid down.

Theme 4: Stability/Continuity

Caregivers speculated that the pets might have provided a sense of stability or continuity for some persons living with dementia, because of their relationships with animals earlier in life. All caregivers reported that their person living with dementia previously had pets. They indicated that their prior relationships with animals was the reason for trying a Joy for All™ pet and/or the reason they believed the person living with dementia responded as they did to the pet. Within their brief responses, we discovered repeated use of specific words denoting positive emotions, for example, "love" was mentioned 20 times, and "happy," six times. One caregiver reported:

> My mother lived next door to me and then when she developed severe dementia, Alzheimer's, I, my husband and I literally moved in with her. Yes, she had two little dogs. And let's see, I even had to give the, the real dogs an interaction with the robotic animals when I brought them into the house. But yeah, I knew I knew it would be of benefit for her since she did love animals.

Other caregivers described relationships the person living with dementia had had with animals earlier in life. As one caregiver shared, "my mother has always had a fondness for dogs of all sizes and breeds . . . My mother has always enjoyed animals but has always had a four-legged companion by her side." A few participants currently had pets that the person living with dementia sometimes interacted with. They explained that the robotic pet was more suitable, citing lack of veterinary bills, toileting and purchasing food as reasons.

Theme 5: Reality Just Might Not Always Matter

Our last theme addresses the criticism in the literature that robotic pets could be infantilizing or, worse, creating additional confusion. While many of the caretakers expressed initial skepticism on the overall effects of a "fake" pet and many reported behaviors by their family member suggesting, at times, that the person did think the robotic pet was real (e.g., feeding the pet, calling the pet to come, directing it to actions), in the end, all expressed an overall positive experience for the person living with dementia. One daughter stated:

> I knew at this stage in her dementia that right now she would know that her Joy for All™ pet dog Dash is robotic. However, Mom gradually seems to be getting more forgetful, and I know that the possibility of her thinking that Dash is alive could one day be a possibility. This fact does not worry me because she has formed such a bond with Dash that I believe he will bring her comfort, unconditional love and companionship as she sleeps until the end of her days here on earth.

In contrast, some participants were sure their person living with dementia realized the robotic pet was not real: "I knew my uncle would notice it was not real, but he did not care because he was excited to have a pet that did not have to go outside, make a mess or go to the vet." The caregivers emphasized that the pet provided comfort and meaning in the lives of the person living with dementia.

Below are suggestions for introducing a person living with dementia to a robotic pet.

Introducing the Robotic Pet

1. Explain how the robotic pet works to the caregiver. Only give the person with dementia as much explanation as they want.
2. Encourage persons under care to name their pets.
3. Show the caregiver how to use the robotic pet because they will usually be the person who will initiate its use. (That includes on/off switches, verbal commands and the location of the batteries).
4. Demonstrate the pets' abilities, so the person under care is not alarmed by the pet's capabilities, adaptabilities, or limitations, especially since many robotic pets respond through verbal and motion reactions and are trained to the voice of the owner.
5. Watch for cues of acceptance or rejection by the person under care. Robotic pets may not be suitable for all persons. Any behaviors denoting fear would need to be addressed. In our observations, one person living with dementia did show fear toward the robotic pet and the pet was removed from the environment. As a preventative, check that the person living with dementia does not have a fear of animals, particularly dogs. However, robotic pets now come in many different animal forms: dogs, cats, birds, even non-animal robots.
6. If the person under care addresses the robotic pet as "real," there is no need to actively dissuade the person.
7. Care for the robotic pet by ensuring it does not get wet, the batteries are fresh, and the machine is charged—so the person does not become agitated if the robotic pet is inoperable.

Here are some activities that will help the robotic pet become part of the routines of persons living with dementia.

Steps to Activity

1. If appropriate, help the person under care voice "train" the pet to its owner.
2. Add identifying tags to the pet designating the owner—especially if the person or persons under care reside in a long-term facility.
3. Share in preparing a space for the pet to be in the person's room or fit on the person's walker, wheelchair, or other special areas.
4. Introduce the pet to others—family, friends, caregivers, other residents and/or staff.
5. Include the pet in routine activities such as mealtime, physical therapy, time in the common areas and/or outings—if possible.
6. Use conversation starters like "How is (pet's name) today?" or "Where would you like to walk with (pet's name)?" or "Where has (robot cat's name) been curled up and sleeping today?" to encourage the person under care to talk about their pet.

Reflection

Our interactions with the caregivers of people living with dementia showed that the *Joy for All*™ robotic pets were appreciated by eight out of the nine persons living with dementia who participated in the study. The pets served as tools for facilitating reminiscence–memories of previous pets and feelings of love and joy related to them–and also validated the person living with dementia's reality and demonstrated that their feelings, thoughts and opinions were acknowledged and respected by the caregiver. Validation therapy is a type of interactive cognitive therapy developed by Feil (1972, 1993, 2017) for use in older adults with cognitive disorders and dementia in which caregivers accept the reality and personal truth of another's experience. Here, the caregivers maintained the interpretations of the persons living with dementia regarding the robotic pets, accepted their preference for conversations with them over humans, and respected their acceptance of the pets as real or not real.

Conclusion

Robotic pets can be a helpful tool for older persons and persons living with dementia. They can be a motivating force enabling people to engage in conversation, to exercise, to participate in therapies—physical or other—and to dine with others. Overall, they can increase the joy of everyday life. Across our sample, caregivers concurred that the pets afforded various benefits for the persons in their care. Chief among these benefits was the love and companionship these pets provided their owners by simply providing someone to talk to. Thus, the results we see from providing a robotic pet, one this book and our individual research agendas look toward, is an increase in overall quality of life for persons living with dementia and their caregivers.

Questions to Consider

1. What do you envision being the greatest benefit to persons living with dementia who are provided with a robotic pet?
2. What, if any, concerns do you have for providing a robotic pet for persons living with dementia?
3. To advocate providing robotic pets for the persons living with dementia in your care (e.g., home, long-term residential facility), write a proposal that provides both sufficient healthcare rationale and a proposed budget to do so.
4. What do you envision being the greatest pushback from family or administration against providing robotic pets? How might you counter these expected issues?
5. How might you facilitate the introduction and acclimation of robotic pets with persons living with dementia?
6. Did this chapter initiate other ideas for improving the quality of life of the persons living with dementia or older persons within your care or you imagine to be in your care?

Resources

1. About companion therapy: www.alzstore.com/doll-pet-therapy-dementia-s/1516.htm?utm_source=google&utm_campaign=Alzheimer%27s+-Priority+-Broad+-+tRoas&utm_medium=ppc&gad_source=1
2. Sale of companion pets: www.alzstore.com/alzheimers-companion-pet-therapy-p/0604.htm?utm_source=google&utm_campaign=Campaign%20-%20PLA%20Shopping&utm_medium=pla&gad_source=1
3. Joy for All™ companion pets: https://joyforall.com/?gclid=Cj0KCQiAkKqsBhC3ARIsAEEjuJh0TahzHnsylIn5Jf1GDtq5R6ls0Zf1jhW6YmMSJWiWSbJEyA9j9EIaAgcFEALw_wcB
4. S. Petersen, S. Houston, H. Qin, C. Tague & J. Studley. (2017). The utilization of robotic pets in dementia care. *Journal of Alzheimer's Disease*, 55(2), 569–574. https://doi.org/10.3233/JAD-160703.

Note

1 In snowball sampling "a random sample of individuals is drawn from a given finite population" (Goodman, 1961, p. 148). It is convenient and "relies on referrals from initially sampled respondents to other persons believed to have the characteristic of interest" (Johnson, 2005, p. 7).
2 Price check is based on a merchandise Internet search as of January 1, 2024, in US dollars.

References

Ambrosi, C., Zaiontz, C., Peragine, G., Sarchi, S., & Bona, F. (2019). Randomized controlled study on the effectiveness of animal-assisted therapy on depression, anxiety, and illness perception in institutionalized elderly. *Psychogeriatrics, 19*(1), 55–64.

Beck, A. M., & Katcher, A. H. (1996). *Between pets and people: The importance of animal companionship*. Purdue University Press.

Bosco, F. M., & Tirassa, M. (2022). Sharedness as an innate basis for communication in the infant. In *Proceedings of the Twentieth Annual Conference of the Cognitive Science Society* (pp. 162–166). Routledge.

Chang, S. J., Lee, J., An, H., Hong, W. H., & Lee, J. Y. (2021). Animal-assisted therapy as an intervention for older adults: A systematic review and meta-analysis to guide evidence-based practice. *Worldviews on Evidence-Based Nursing, 18*(1), 60–67.

Clare, L., & Shakespeare, P. (2004). Negotiating the impact of forgetting: Dimensions of resistance in task-oriented conversations between people with early-stage dementia and their partners. *Dementia, 3*(2), 211–232.

Coghlan, D. (2021). Fostering undergraduate research through insider inquiry: Exploiting student work experiences. *Management Teaching Review, 6*(1), 66–72. https://doi.org/10.1177/2379298119855747

Davis, B. H. (Ed.). (2005). Alzheimer talk, text and context: Enhancing communication. Palgrave Macmillan.

Davis, B., Maclagan, M., & Pope, C. (2021). Digital outreach in online dementia discourse: A preliminary introduction. *Journal of Interactional Research in Communication Disorders, 12*(2), 185–211. https://doi.org/10.1558/jircd.22571

Feil, N. (1972). A new approach to group therapy with the senile psychotic aged. *Gerontological Society*, Winter Conference. San Juan.

Feil, N. (1993). The validation breakthrough: Simple techniques for communicating with people with "Alzheimer's-type dementia." Health Promotion Press.

Feil, N. (2017). Validation therapy. In *Serving the elderly* (pp. 89–116). Routledge.

Goodman, L. A. (1961). Snowball sampling. *The Annals of Mathematical Statistics, 30*(1), 148–170.

Guendouzi, J. A., & Müller, N. (2006). *Approaches to discourse in dementia*. Lawrence Erlbaum Associates.

Hamilton, H. E. (1994). *Conversations with an Alzheimer's patient: An interactional sociolinguistic study.* Cambridge University Press.

Hamilton, H. E. (2011). At the intersection of art, Alzheimer's disease, and discourse: Talk in the surround of paintings. In P. Backhaus (Ed.), *Communication in elderly care: Cross-cultural approaches* (pp. 166–193). Continuum.

Hudson, J., Ungar, R., Albright, L., Tkatch, R., Schaeffer, J., & Wicker, E. R. (2020). Robotic pet use among community-dwelling older adults. *The Journals of Gerontology. Series B, Psychological Sciences and Social Sciences, 75*(9), 2018–2028. https://doi.org/10.1093/geronb/gbaa119

Isaac, A. R., & Hamilton, H. E. (2020). Meaningfulness at the intersection of knowledge and environmental objects: Investigating interactions in art galleries and residences involving persons living with dementia and their carers. In T. Stickle (Ed.) *Learning from the talk of persons living with dementia: A practical guide to interaction and interactional research* (pp. 135–163). Springer Nature.

Johnson, T. P. (2005). Snowball sampling. In *Encyclopedia of biostatistics* (p. 7). Wiley. https://doi.org/10.1002/0470011815.b2a16070

Kirk, R. G., Pemberton, N., & Quick, T. (2019). Being well together? promoting health and well-being through more than human collaboration and companionship. *Medical Humanities, 45*(1), 75–81. https://doi.org/10.1136/medhum-2018-011601.

Matsumoto, Y. (2011). Painful to playful: Quotidian frames in the conversational discourse of older Japanese speakers. *Language in Society, 40*(5), 591–616. https://doi.org/10.1017/S0047404511000698

Matsumoto, Y. (2019). Taking the stance of quotidian in talking about pains: Resilience and defiance. *Linguistics Vanguard, 5*(s2). https://doi.org/10.1515/lingvan-2018-0034

Ramanathan, V. (1997). *Alzheimer discourse: Some sociolinguistic dimensions.* Lawrence Erlbaum Associates.

Ryan, E. B., Byrne, K., Spykerman, H., & Orange, J. B. (2005). Evidencing Kitwood's personhood strategies: Conversation as care in dementia. In B. H. Davis (Ed.), *Alzheimer talk, text and context: Enhancing communication* (pp. 190–198). Palgrave Macmillan.

Santhanaraj, K., Ramya, M., & Dinkaran, D. (2021). A survey of assistive robots and systems for elderly care. *Journal of Enabling Technologies, 15*(1), 66–72. https://doi.org/10.1108/JET-10-2020-0043

Stickle, T. (2023). Conversation practices that foster or hinder inclusivity during interactions involving persons living with dementia. *Pragmatics and Society, 15*(1), 196–213. https://doi.org/10.1075/ps.23052.sti

Troutman-Jordan, M. (2021). Interdisciplinary collaboration for experiential learning in gerontology research. https://teaching.charlotte.edu/teaching-transformation/sotl-grants-program.

Van Assche, M., Petrovic, M., Cambier, D., Calders, P., Van Gelder, P., & Van de Velde, D. (2022). The perspectives of older adults with mild cognitive impairment and their caregivers on the use of socially assistive robots in healthcare: Exploring factors that influence attitude in a pre-implementation stage. *Disability and Rehabilitation. Assistive Technology*, 19(1), 222–232. https://doi.org/10.1080/17483107.202 2.2075477

Vercelli, A., Rainero, I., Ciferri, L., Boido, M., & Pirri, F. (2017). Robots in elderly care. *DigiCult | Scientific Journal on Digital Cultures*, 2(2), 37–50. https://doi.org/10.4399/97888255088954

Appendix

Interview Questions

1. Did you choose a Joy for All™ dog or a cat?
2. Did you previously have a real dog or cat at home? How about now?
3. What kinds of things did your loved one do with the robotic pet?
4. Did the person hug, pet, snuggle or love on it?
5. Did the person whisper or talk to it or call it by a name?
6. What effect do you think the pet had on the person's speech, mood or behavior?
7. And what has been your overall reaction to this robot pet?
8. Did it ever worry you that your loved one might think the new pet was truly alive?
9. Did you have any other worries or concerns about the new pet? If so, please describe.
10. If you have any other thoughts or opinions about the use of robotic pets with persons living with dementia, would you please share these?

11 Conclusion

Lorna E. Segall and Trini Stickle

Introduction

The authors hope that by reading all or parts of this collection, you, the reader, will feel empowered, inspired, and supported in providing a variety of caregiving activities. Each chapter in this text is highly relevant, offering adaptable and feasible strategies for a wide range of populations and needs. We hope these ideas create opportunities that transcend traditional caregiving roles that foster genuine, person to person engagement where the disease becomes almost irrelevant. We anticipate that the information shared in these chapters finds its way into working with populations beyond persons with dementia. Many of these activities are excellent engagement strategies for those with autism, residing in foster care, recovering from trauma, and many more. For example, Voices in Motion (Chapter 7) could be employed with Parkinson's patients and their caregivers, or on family visitation days at prisons. Commonplace books (Chapter 4) could be a way for children in foster homes, or those incarcerated to share their stories. Bingocize® (Chapter 8) could be incorporated with children learning body awareness or learning to follow directions and adults who may be experiencing mild movement disorders or in a rehabilitation setting would benefit from this intervention. We believe that our readers will find other ways to apply, alter, or create additional activities inspired by the ones housed in this volume to enhance the lives of others.

What We Have Learned

Each chapter showcases the potential of individuals, regardless of their diagnosis, and highlights the caregiver's ability to create meaningful moments in diverse ways with evidence-based approaches. We've explored the impact of intergenerational engagement with persons with dementia and how each of these interventions can be modified to fit a variety of settings, resources, and populations. We've demonstrated

DOI: 10.4324/9781003359463-13

how incorporating these activities with students enhances their knowledge of the human experience and prepares them as future caregiving professionals and as the future of aging. For example, the AIR program (Chapter 6) illustrates how not only the residents and AIRs benefitted from the intergenerational engagement, but also the staff, administrators, and family members. Through the art of haiku making (Chapter 5), participants mutually engage in creative self-expression through equal participation. For many of us, creating haiku poems is a new experience and allows the caregiver and the care receiver to learn something new together. Collaborating with the power of technology (Chapter 10) through animatronics to support and supplement the work of humans is explored as an innovative approach to harnessing connection. Notably, the activities presented in these chapters can enhance all forms of human interaction, even in the absence of any disease and reminds us that everyone can engage. We believe the accessibility of the humanities levels the playing field and allows us to interact regardless of disease, ability, or resources. By meeting care receivers where they are, caregivers can provide what their patients need and help themselves, too. By employing intergenerational connections, we can counteract many of today's most urgent needs of aging, foremost the detrimental consequences of isolation and loneliness. Arguably, the lack of social engagement or, rather, the physical and mental detriment that results from it, is an epidemic affecting us all. As such, it is a problem in need of amelioration. To that end, we attempt to re-write the aging journey by starting with young people.

From Research to Activities to Education

Normalizing the incorporation of the humanities within the caregiving space begins in the classroom with our future caregivers. Below we offer innovative curricular ideas for various types of educational applications.

Clinical Curricula

In medical programs, already dense with credit hours, practicums, and requirements, it is essential to make space for patient-centered engagement that is not solely focusing on the diagnosis. This raises the question of how to meaningfully accomplish this curricular modification within the existing parameters of credit hours. Medical humanities–the use of lessons from literature, art, music, and such–could be expanded to incorporate the reciprocity of learning by teaching the types of activities present within this volume, where students in caregiving degree programs benefit from knowledge shared with students in medical degree programs. The reciprocal learning experiences could be woven into existing coursework through guest lectures, video or audio data, or group learning experiences. Identifying the needs of student interaction should further be tailored to various specialties.

Fostering connections with geriatric medical specialties can highlight the role of humanities in patient care. Discussion of case studies, co-treatment practices, or interdisciplinary discussion would offer meaningful perspective into each discipline. Collaborative learning experiences can be particularly valuable, involving partnerships with related departments such as Science and Brain Health, Psychology of Aging, and Social Work with a focus on Aging and Dementia (Paris et al., 2021; Templeman et al., 2016). Furthermore, exploring the role of the arts in aging care and the hospital setting, including music and creative writing, can provide significant benefits. Participation in these activities as a student with an older adult is impactful to underscoring the value of these interventions. The objective through these experiences is to not only create a human centered approach to care, but to also develop an understanding and appreciation for related disciplines and to empower them for one another. Maybe, instead of, or, in addition to, a patient receiving medication for loneliness or isolation, a physician could recommend and offer community resources that offer creative writing or music, for example.

Undergraduate Health Care and Social Work Curriculum

Examining topics at the intersection of health, care, and geriatric services, such as appropriate care, dignity in care, affirming care, and policies affecting aging individuals would offer a well-rounded foundation for undergraduate students. Collaborating with interdisciplinary colleagues to create shared learning experiences and foster reciprocal knowledge benefits all learners, including instructors. Advocating for healthcare professionals to appreciate the humanities' contributions is vital, as is ensuring that care-focused degree programs gain a comprehensive understanding of the healthcare system and its impact on patient care from a medical professional's perspective.

Partnerships of this type of aging-related coursework could include aging studies, social work with aging populations, social health, and brain health sciences, while also addressing health disparities among aging demographics. For undergraduate students, presenting these ideas highlights the importance of professional collaboration and encourages them to consider the biopsychosocial implications of each human's experience. These approaches achieve deeper, genuine human engagement, shifting the traditional roles of patient and caregiver to a more human to human interaction.

Undergraduate General Education Curriculum and Experience

Understanding and interacting with older adults extends beyond clinical, medical, and caregiving degrees. Given the projected growth of the aging population in the U.S. and the world, it would seem important for all students to develop a greater awareness and engagement with the aging demographic. Regardless of the degree program, learning opportunities with the aging population influences not only their personal development and well-being but also enhances their professional competencies across various fields.

Professions across the spectrum benefit from intergenerational coursework. While it is clear why professions like attorneys or educators benefit from knowing more about older adults, it is also important, and maybe less obvious, for engineering students to understand the needs of an aging population for whom they may be developing assistive products for (Czaja & Sharit, 2009). Similarly, financial planners would be better prepared for supporting clients in the cost of funding assisted living and working with clients experiencing early stages of cognitive decline (Vien, 2017).

Healthy aging is a valuable topic for people of all ages. Including young people in discussions about healthy aging can begin to reshape the aging narrative and how we age in the future. For undergraduate students, it is valuable to create opportunities for interaction with older adults. Not all, but many young adults find interacting with older adults, particularly those with dementia, intimidating. Early, simple engagement experiences can demystify these interactions and build confidence, allowing for more complex engagements later.

For educators introducing their students to the aging population, it is advantageous to consider that the experiences of young adults with older adults vary widely. Some students may have close relationships with their grandparents while others may not have known their grandparents at all. In some cases, this may be their first significant loss of a loved one. These differences, along with their current stage in life and grief processing, should be considered for classroom experiences to be meaningful. It is essential to align learning objectives with the developmental stage of young adults to maximize the benefits of this engagement. Initiating a brief student survey at the beginning of each semester or even sharing this perspective during class orientations would prepare students and faculty members for a productive experience. These steps also allow any additional preparation or modifications to be made. Staying mindful of these factors ensures that young adults gain valuable insights and skills from their interactions with the older population that they can carry forward in their future professional and personal lives.

Changing the Ways We Care

Caregiving isn't prescriptive and is best designed to meet the needs of the individual considered separately from the diagnosis. There is no one way to best care for any individual regardless of diagnosis. The idiosyncratic nature of human beings is reflected in their response to illness and refusal to acknowledge this perspective and incorporate it into our care does not allow us to best care for those in need. Particularly for persons with dementia whose previous life experiences are so intricately woven into their dementia experience, we must focus on humanity, to most effectively meet their needs. The partnership between medicine and the humanities is a direct line to treating not only the person but also supporting and empowering the caregiver. This is an exciting opportunity to change the way we care by incorporating humanities-based practices early in the future of health professionals' learning. Through coursework, experiential learning activities, and collaborations with humanities informed coursework, we can begin including humanities-based approaches for our future medical providers.

For Elderly

It is the authors' aim to emphasize that persons with dementia are, first and foremost, people, regardless of their diagnosis. We hope the ideas presented here inspire you to focus on a person's abilities rather than the challenges posed by their condition or diagnosis. The chapters present a range of resources, time commitments, and materials, along with modifications and suggestions for achieving the same objectives through different approaches and materials. We encourage you to apply these insights to other populations as well as those with dementia.

Local

While every community differs in resources, nearly all are intergenerational. Identifying the specific opportunities and resources in each community to connect generations can inspire innovative and exciting collaborations that benefit all members and enhance overall wellbeing. To expand the impact, sharing these experiences within your network and neighborhoods provides a platform for offering inspiration, encouraging participation, and presenting new ideas. Whether you are part of a bustling metropolis, a college town, or a rural area, opportunities exist. Earlier, we discussed the challenges posed by COVID-19, and we've seen that where there's a will, there's a way. Although we touched on the negative impacts of social media on wellbeing, it can also be a powerful and efficient tool for sharing experiences with both our local communities and the broader world.

Global

Loneliness and isolation among the aging population are not unique to the United States. Globally, and across all age groups, the epidemic of isolation is evident, affecting many (Surkalim et al., 2022). Feelings of inclusion and social connectedness are fundamental to the human experience and are directly linked to mental and physical health for all ages (Shah & Househ, 2023). For example, children and adolescents who report positive relationships with parents, teachers, and friends tend to perform better academically and have better mental health (DuBois et al., 2011; Prizeman, Weinstein & McCabe, 2023). For older adults who maintain active social networks or live in retirement communities, the impacts of isolation and loneliness may be mitigated. For those who may be limited due to mobility, illness, or resources, isolation and loneliness can have severe impacts on wellbeing. Even common age-related milestones such as retirement or the loss of friends, are important when considering how loneliness plays a role in wellbeing (Valtorta & Hanratty, 2012). Moreover, the stigma associated with loneliness may prevent individuals from seeking help and receiving necessary services (Prizeman, Weinstein & McCabe, 2023). In many communities, the fear of rejection and societal exclusion often leads to further isolation and loneliness.

Disadvantaged

Many of the most marginalized communities in our society experience the highest rates of loneliness and isolation (Rogan, 2024). Groups such as LGBTQIA+, BIPOC, immigrants, returning servicemen, and those in lower socioeconomic communities are particularly at risk for these feelings of isolation (Garcia et al., 2019; McGuire et al., 2023; Rogan, 2024).

The chapters in this text provide meaningful ways to share diverse perspectives that can be implemented at various levels. Humanities-inspired activities offer creative, feasible, relatable, and approachable methods of engagement and expression, facilitating easy rapport building. For example, a young adult in the LGBTQIA+ community might share experiences related to self-identity and feelings of insecurity through a commonplace book. Similarly, a cohort of returning servicemen could find camaraderie by singing in a choir, while a group of refugee children might relay their immigration experiences to their citizen peers through letter writing, storytelling, or postcard exchanges. When we engage with someone seemingly different from ourselves, commonalities quickly become evident and are amplified through these person-centered opportunities for connection.

Persons Living with Dementia

Chronic isolation and loneliness, or even the perception of these feelings, in older adults can increase the risk of developing dementia by 50% (Lazzari & Rabattini, 2016; Yang et al., 2016). The profound impact of intergenerational engagement with this community is transformative, significantly improving the wellbeing of individuals and their caregivers grappling with this disease. Managing dementia is extraordinarily challenging, requiring immense patience, and perseverance, often when both patients and caregivers are already exhausted. Yet, within these moments of frustration and perceived impossibility, lie opportunities to connect, communicate, and be heard. These moments transcend where the humanities go beyond the diagnosis and highlight the power of our shared community.

Persons in Prison

The aging population within America's prison system is one of the fastest growing and costliest demographics (Kaiksow et al., 2023). Many incarcerated older adults suffer from physical and mental health issues, such as dementia, often exacerbated by years of stress and trauma (Kaiksow et al., 2023). As a result, aging inmates require additional care for activities of daily living due to physical or cognitive impairments (NCCHC, 2024). Lack of resources, trained care, and functional living conditions make aging in the prison system particularly difficult.

The challenges faced by aging inmates extend beyond their time in prison. Upon release, additional social support services and community resources are crucial for the challenging process of successful reintegration, which are often difficult to access (NCCHC, 2024). Aging inmates are perhaps the most secluded and isolated group, at high risk of needing extensive care, yet having access to the fewest resources. Furthermore, they often receive little to no social empathy due to ageism and the stigma surrounding incarceration.

Even if you never set foot in a prison as a caregiver, you are likely to interact with someone who has been incarcerated or someone with a loved one impacted by the justice system. Most currently incarcerated individuals will eventually be released and return to society. Understanding these challenges can foster a more empathetic and supportive community for all.

For Others

Caregiving for a loved one with dementia presents substantial challenges. Considering that a lifetime of memories and experiences have been shared, witnessing the cognitive decline of a friend or family member can be devastating. Caregivers experience tremendous stress, often leading to burnout, isolation, and causing caregivers to sacrifice their own health and wellbeing (Lorig et al., 2019). Although numerous resources are available to support caregivers in maintaining their health and well-being, the risk of isolation and loneliness remains high (Cochran et al., 2022; Massimo et al., 2023; Lynn, 2022; Alzheimer's Association, n.d.; National Institute on Aging, 2024). Current research also indicates that engaging in shared activities with persons with dementia can alleviate caregiver burnout (Petrovsky et al., 2024; Gitlin et al., 2021). These shared meaning-making interactions frequently result in meaningful and tangible artifacts.

Caregivers come in many forms to include spouses, nurses, CNAs, social workers, administrators, teachers, and neighbors. Their experience and wellbeing is crucial in maintaining the wellbeing of everyone in their care. Just as many are reluctant to admit to experiencing feelings of loneliness and isolation, caregivers, too, can be hesitant to seek help, or feel guilty for needing additional support. Their role must not be neglected and each of these chapters plays a role in supporting the caregiver.

The activities outlined in this book are designed to be creative and enjoyable, producing thoughtful products worth sharing in the community and the classroom. Sharing the outcomes of these interventions beyond the caregiving space and into the community and the classroom could broaden their scope of impact. In this scenario, not only would the engagement of participating in these activities offer meaningful interaction for caregivers and persons living with dementia, but they would also aid in redefining societal perceptions of what aging and caregiving look like. Imagine seeing haiku poetry created by persons with dementia featured in a local magazine or dementia choirs performing at professional or collegiate concerts. Such initiatives can help make the topics of caregiving and dementia more approachable and engaging, fostering productive conversations around these often-avoided subjects. Because we are all aging, these discussions are pertinent to everyone. It also serves as a platform for building community in this space, and moves the concept of and changes during aging to be part of our discussion of all ages, not just the elderly (or the very young).

The growing issue of isolation and loneliness affects all age groups, exacerbated in an era where social media often replaces direct human contact. This social media shift has diminished the frequency and quality of meaningful connections. However, when used thoughtfully, technology and social media can actually enhance connectivity, as demonstrated during the COVID-19 pandemic. Despite physical separation, technology allowed us to see and hear each other, maintaining essential human connections.

While we may never fully escape the threat of future pandemics requiring the need for extended isolation, one key lesson from the recent crisis is that caregiving thrives where perseverance meets creativity. With this understanding, we can strive to make the final years of anyone's life both meaningful and valuable.

References

Alzheimer's Association. (n.d.) Be a health caregiver. www.alz.org/help-support/caregiving/caregiverhealth/be_a_healthy_caregiver

Cochran, F. A., Paun, O., Strayhorn, S., & Barnes, L. L. (2022). 'Walk a mile in my shoes:' African American caregiver perceptions of caregiving and self-care. *Ethnicity & Health*, 27(2), 435–452. https://doi.org/10.1080/13557858.2020.1734777

Czaja, S.J. & Sharit, J. (2009). The aging of the population: Opportunities and challenges for human factors engineering. *The Bridge: Linking Engineering and Society*, 39(1), 34–40.

DuBois, D. L., Portillo, N., Rhodes, J. E., Silverthorn, N., & Valentine, J. C. (2011). How effective are mentoring programs for youth? A systematic assessment of the evidence. *Psychological Science in the Public Interest: A Journal of the American Psychological Society*, 12(2), 57–91. https://doi.org/10.1177/1529100611414806

Garcia, J., Vargas, N., Clark, J. L., Magaña Álvarez, M., Nelons, D. A., & Parker, R. G. (2019). Social isolation and connectedness as determinants of well-being: Global evidence mapping focused on LGBTQ youth. *Global Public Health*, 15(4), 497–519. https://doi.org/10.1080/17441692.2019.1682028

Gitlin, L. N., Marx, K., Piersol, C. V., Hodgson, N. A., Huang, J., Roth, D. L., & Lyketsos, C. (2021). Effects of the tailored activity program (TAP) on dementia-related symptoms, health events and caregiver well being: A randomized controlled trial. *BMC Geriatrics*, 21(1), 581. https://doi.org/10.1186/s12877-021-02511-4

Kaiksow, F. A., Brown, L., & Merss, K. B. (2023). Caring for the rapidly aging incarcerated population: The role of policy. *Journal of Gerontological Nursing*, 49(3), 7–11. https://doi.org/10.3928/00989134-20230209-02

Lazzari, C., & Rabottini, M. (2022). COVID-19, loneliness, social isolation and risk of dementia in older people: A systematic review and meta-analysis of the relevant literature. *International Journal of Psychiatry in Clinical Practice*, 26(2), 196–207. https://doi.org/10.1080/13651501.2021.1959616

Lorig, K., Ritter, P. L., Laurent, D. D., & Yank, V. (2019). Building better caregivers: A pragmatic 12-Month trial of a community-based workshop for caregivers of cognitively impaired adults. *Journal of Applied Gerontology*, 38(9), 1228–1252. https://doi.org/10.1177/0733464817741682

Lynn, A. (2022). The criticality of self-care by dementia caregivers. www.americanbar.org/groups/senior_lawyers/resources/voice-of-experience/2010-2022/criticality-self-care-dementia-caregivers/

McGuire, A. P., Elmore, C., Szabo, Y. Z., Kurz, A. S., Mendoza, C., Umucu, E., & Creech, S. K. (2023). Exploring the trajectory and correlates of social isolation for veterans across a 6-month period during COVID-19. *PloS one*, 18(3), e0281575. https://doi.org/10.1371/journal.pone.0281575

Massimo, L., Hirschman, K. B., Aryal, S., Quinn, R., Fisher, L., Sharkey, M., Thomas, G., Bowles, K. H., & Riegel, B. (2023). iCare4Me for FTD: A pilot randomized study to improve self-care in caregivers of persons with frontotemporal degeneration. *Alzheimer's & Dementia: Translational Research & Clinical Interventions*, 9(2). https://doi.org/10.1002/trc2.12381

National Institute on Aging. (n.d.) Alzheimer's caregiving: Caring for yourself. www.nia.nih.gov/health/alzheimers-caregiving/alzheimers-caregiving-caring-yourself

NCCHC. (2024). Care for Aging Patients in the Correctional Setting: A position statement. www.ncchc.org/position-statements/care-for-aging-patients-in-the-correctional-setting/

Paris, D. M., Guest, H., Winckler, D., Slaymaker, R., East, K., & Baldridge, S. (2021). Collaboration in medicine: The role of interprofessional education. *Journal of Evidence-Based Social Work*, 18(5), 527–533. https://doi.org/10.1080/26408066.2021.1919273

Petrovsky, D. V., Yildiz, M., Yefimova, M., Sefcik, J. S., Baker, Z. G., Ma, K. P. K., Rahemi, Z., Bacsu, J.-D. R., Smith, M. L., Pickering, C. E. Z., & Leggett, A. N. (2024). Shared activities as a protective factor against behavioral and psychological symptoms of dementia and caregiver stress. *Innovation in Aging*, 8(5). https://doi.org/10.1093/geroni/igae034

Prizeman, K., Weinstein, N., & McCabe, C. (2023). Effects of mental health stigma on loneliness, social isolation, and relationships in young people with depression symptoms. *BMC Psychiatry*, 23(1), 527. https://doi.org/10.1186/s12888-023-04991-7

Rogan, A. (February 24, 2024). How a growing crisis of loneliness is affecting Americans' health. www.pbs.org/newshou/show/how-a-growing-crisis-of-loneliness-is-affecting-americans-health

Shah, H. A., & Househ, M. (2023). Understanding loneliness in younger people: Review of the opportunities and challenges for loneliness interventions. *Interactive Journal of Medical Research*, 12, e45197. https://doi.org/10.2196/45197

Surkalim, D. L., Luo, M., Eres, R., Gebel, K., van Buskirk, J., Bauman, A., & Ding, D. (2022). The prevalence of loneliness across 113 countries: Systematic review and meta-analysis. *BMJ, 376,* e067068. https://doi.org/10.1136/bmj-2021-067068

Templeman, K., Robinson, A. & McKenna, L. (2016). Advancing medical education: Connecting interprofessional collaboration and education opportunities with integrative medicine initiatives to build shared learning. *Journal of Complementary and Integrative Medicine, 13*(4), 347–355. https://doi-org.echo.louisville.edu/10.1515/jcim-2016-0002

Valtorta, N., & Hanratty, B. (2012). Loneliness, isolation and the health of older adults: Do we need a new research agenda?. *Journal of the Royal Society of Medicine, 105*(12), 518–522. https://doi.org/10.1258/jrsm.2012.120128

Vien, C. L. (2017). What all CPAs should know about elder planning. *Journal of Accountancy, 224*(1), 46–50.

Yang, Y. C., Boen, C., Gerken, K., Li, T., Schorpp, K., & Harris, K. M. (2016). Social relationships and physiological determinants of longevity across the human lifespan. *Proceedings of the National Academy of Sciences of the United States of America, 113*(3), 578–583. https://doi.org/10.1073/pnas.1511085112

Glossary

ableism   Discrimination in favor of persons who are able-bodied.

activities of daily living (ADLs)   Basic tasks people do for self-care, such as eating, dressing, bathing, and grooming.

ageism   Discrimination on the basis of age.

agency   The feeling of ownership of one's actions and responsibility for them.

animatronic   The use of machines controlled by computer software to make puppets, models, or other inanimate objects move in a natural way.

artifact   An object made by a human being, typically an item of cultural or historical interest.

Beautiful Questions   Open-ended prompts that help spark the imagination, e.g., "If love were an object, what would it be?"

bingo   A game in which players match numbered squares on a card with numbers called out until someone wins by matching certain squares.

Bingocize®   A socially engaging group-based program that combines exercise, health education, and the widely popular game of bingo.

cognitive pragmatics   The study of communication as a cooperative activity through which participants consciously and intentionally construct the meaning.

commonplace book   The literary practice of gathering and organizing fragments from different texts and miscellaneous excerpts deemed to be useful, wise, or otherwise memorable in abstracted forms.

commonplacing (v.)   To gather and organize fragments from different texts and miscellaneous excerpts deemed to be useful, wise, or otherwise memorable in abstract forms.

coronary event   The term cardiac event is used to denote the composite of a variety of adverse events related to the cardiovascular system.

COVID-19   coronavirus disease 2019; a disease caused by a virus named SARS-CoV-2.

dementia   A general term for neurocognitive diseases which cause loss of memory, language, problem-solving and other thinking abilities that are severe enough to interfere with daily life.

Global North   Refers to the relative power and wealth of countries in distinct parts of the world, presently North America, Europe, and Australia.

haiku   A 17-syllable poetic form originating in Japan.

health humanities   The intersection of health and humanistic disciplines (such as philosophy, religion, literature) and fine arts, as well as social science research (such as history, anthropology, sociology, and cultural studies) in patient care.

health literacy   The ability of individuals to obtain and translate knowledge and information in order to maintain and improve one's health.

intergenerational   Existing or occurring between or among persons of different generations.

intergenerational programming   Existing or occurring between or among persons of different generations.

medical humanities   A field of study that contextualizes what it means to be human as part of health and healthcare; a holistic approach to medical education that unites the arts, humanities, and social sciences to address persons suffering from illness or injury first from as a human being.

medico-therapeutics   A branch of medical science dealing with the application of remedies to diseases.

mild cognitive impairment (MCI)   Declines in thinking, memory, language, and judgment that can occur during the aging process before more serious decline resulting from dementia.

Mini Mental State Examination   A set of 11 questions that doctors and other healthcare professionals commonly use to check for cognitive impairment, i.e., problems with thinking, communication, understanding and memory.

personhood   The essential characteristics that define being human.

premature death/mortality   Unconditional probability of death between ages 30 and 70 years from cardiovascular diseases, cancer, diabetes, and chronic respiratory diseases.

stroke   Medical incident when blood flow to the brain is blocked (ischemic stroke) or there is sudden bleeding in the brain (hemorrhagic stroke).

suicide ideation   Term used to describe a range of contemplations, wishes, and preoccupations with death and suicide.

Takotsubo cardiomyopathy   A weakening of the left ventricle, the heart's main pumping chamber. The condition is usually the result of severe emotional or physical stress, such as a sudden illness, the loss of a loved one, a serious accident or a natural disaster. Considering the health condition has been linked to emotional events, it is also called broken-heart syndrome.

Voices in Motion™ (ViM)   An intergenerational community-based choir for persons living with dementia, their care partners, and students.

Index